Like It Is

Like It Is

A Teen SEX Guide

by E. James Lieberman, M.D., *and*
Karen Lieberman Troccoli

With best wishes and Thanks for helping calm the hysteria in Montgomery County today— E James Lieberman 11/12/04

McFarland & Company, Inc., Publishers
Jefferson, North Carolina, and London

Pictured on cover: Zack Lawless and Ashley Wagoner
(photograph by Barry Greene).

Drawings by Jennifer M. Leong.

British Library Cataloguing-in-Publication data are available

Library of Congress Cataloguing-in-Publication Data

Lieberman, E. James, 1934–
    Like it is : a teen sex guide / by E. James Lieberman and
Karen Lieberman Troccoli.
       p. cm.
    Includes bibliographical references and index.
    Summary : Provides information about sex, relationships,
and birth control, with an emphasis on informed consent and
mutual respect, and discusses such options as parenthood,
adoption, and abortion.
      ISBN 0-7864-0526-0 (sewn softcover : 50# alkaline paper) ∞
    1. Sex instruction for teenagers.   [1. Sex instruction for
youth.] I. Troccoli, Karen Lieberman. II. Title.
HQ35.L543   1998
613.9'07 — dc21   98-27176
                                            CIP
                                            AC

Manufactured in the United States of America

McFarland & Company, Inc., Publishers
  Box 611, Jefferson, North Carolina 28640

This book is an expression of faith
in the readiness of young people
to govern their futures wisely.
We dedicate it to them,
and to their parents, teachers and counselors.

Acknowledgments

Our experiences with peers and patients, teachers and students, family and friends, form the basis of this book. We owe special thanks to Lisa Kaeser of the Alan Guttmacher Institute, and Debra Hauser and Jane Norman of Advocates for Youth, who reviewed the final draft. Many teens helped formally and informally by sharing their experiences, ideas, insights and questions with us. Jennifer M. Leong provided the illustrations. To Dr. Robert A. Hatcher at Emory University we express admiration and gratitude for his longstanding leadership in family planning education and service. We are heavily indebted to his *Contraceptive Technology* and his work on emergency contraception.

While we take responsibility for any omissions or errors in this book, we remind readers that a book, no matter how accurate, cannot substitute for a visit to the doctor or family planning clinic.

We thank our families, Carol Lieberman and Kenneth and Nicholas Troccoli, for their loving support and always helpful opinions and suggestions along the way.

Table of Contents

Introduction

Every year millions of young Americans discover something new about life from their own bodies. They find out that no matter how much they thought they knew about sex, they have a lot to learn. Unfortunately many learn the hard way, from painful and costly mistakes. We hope that this book will help prevent some of those unhappy experiences.

Parents mean well in their efforts to teach their children about sex, but they often meet a wall of privacy or embarrassment that is quite normal in families at this stage. Teachers may be well prepared, but often they are forbidden to teach certain topics by principals or school boards.

Few teens get advice on sex and contraception from a doctor or nurse. Too often, young women first get family planning information after a pregnancy scare or unplanned pregnancy. The media are full of sexual drama but rarely offer help with sexual realities. Despite its apparent openness, American society leaves young people to fend for themselves in a sexually overheated environment where the cost of mistakes is terribly high. The facts, as of 1995:

• About half of all teenagers — 55 percent of men and 50 percent of women — have intercourse before the age of 20.

• One million adolescent women become pregnant each year.

• Four-fifths (82 percent) of teen pregnancies are unintended.

• Almost half — over 300,000 — of these unintended pregnancies end in abortion.

• Teen mothers are less likely to finish high school.

• One out of four sexually experienced teens contracts a sexually transmitted disease each year; HIV infection is often contracted before age 20.

• Most teens believe the average young person does not have enough accurate information about sex and reproduction.

Sex can be like a roller-coaster ride or like boating on a gentle current. Roller coasters and boats can be quite safe or dangerous, depending on their quality and the circumstances. You would not want to ride a roller coaster that failed inspection by qualified engineers, and you shouldn't go out on a boat without a life preserver. Many lives have been harmed by the pursuit of pleasure without care. Our purpose in this book is to prevent harm by providing guidance to young people who have thoughts and feelings about sex, who will be making decisions affecting their whole lives.

Experts in sex therapy — the treatment of sexual problems — say that "the sexual organs are located between the ears," meaning that the mind, the personality, and one's knowledge and attitudes are more important than the physical "equipment" located below the neck. Young adults, and older ones too, confront emotional, intellectual, and moral questions about sex that have more to do with the mental than the physical side of life. When is a person mature enough to have sex? Is premarital sex ever okay? Is the main purpose of sex to make babies? To have fun? To express love? How can I resist pressure to have sex? What makes sex safe or unsafe? Why do some of my friends take so many chances, as though nothing bad could happen to them, while others are totally afraid?

These kinds of questions have many answers. Sometimes there is only one right answer, but more often there are several. A right answer for one person may be wrong for another. By the same token, answers lead to many different consequences. We wrote this book to help you think about sexual truths and consequences. Where the facts are known, we state them as clearly as possible. Even so, the implications of plain facts are as different as people themselves — depending, for example, on their moral and spiritual values.

These values are being formed at the same time decisions about sexuality have to be made. Religion, morals, relationships, emotions, hormones, and psychology all characterize the complicated stage we call adolescence. Each person tries to weave these themes into a stable, sensible way of being, a personal philosophy or "tapestry" of personality.

This book is a tool for young adults coming to terms with sexuality. It provides a straightforward discussion of the issues while leaving room for readers to decide what is best for themselves. The information is presented with authority, the attitudes with humility. Rarely will everyone have the same judgment in an area as diverse, dynamic and personal as sexual behavior. We speak out on a few matters on which we feel strongly, we give several answers on most issues, and we leave some things entirely to the reader. Our values will be at odds with those of some people. Our goal is to help you be successful in your commitment to the values you cherish.

The stories about young people in this book come from many sources. Sometimes we combine cases to make a point clear. We always change names and identifying details so as not to violate anyone's privacy.

We are concerned with three sexual consequences to be avoided: unintended pregnancy, sexually transmitted disease, and emotional harm resulting from premature intimacy or abusive relationships. That's why this book addresses pregnancy, protection against sexually transmitted diseases, and building sound, healthy relationships.

Because the field is changing rapidly, readers must check with a health professional regarding any personal medical questions, diagnosis or treatment. For updates on general topics and advances see the Resources section. Current information is always available through libraries, reputable organizations, and the Internet, as we indicate.

Much of life's tragedy stems from ignorance, not evil-doers. Young people in particular are often poorly informed and lack access to contraceptive services. Some people say teenagers are too immature to be educated about these things. Others say, "Better a year too soon than an hour too late." We think the problem is too much ignorance about one of the major forces in life. Sex is ancient and modern, private and public, intimate and vast. It includes science, poetry, religion, politics, art, economics ... almost everything we know and do.

Parents are the most important teachers. They teach by example. They impart values along with basic information about sexuality but cannot be expected to deal with all the technical questions that arise. This book is an expression of faith in the readiness of young people to govern their futures wisely. We hope it will be useful to them and their parents, as well as to teachers, librarians and health professionals.

E. James Lieberman, M.D., M.P.H.
Karen Lieberman Troccoli, M.P.H.

Chapter 1

The Many Virtues
and Seven Sins
of Close Relationships

Sow an act and you reap a habit;
sow a habit and you reap a character;
sow a character and you reap a destiny.

What we *choose* to do — what we sow, the quotation reminds us — influences everything: our habits, our personalities, and the society we live in. This chapter looks at choices in close relationships, including sexual ones. Closeness, or intimacy, is one of life's great gifts. Good sex strengthens relationships, but bad sex harms them. This chapter is about relationships, their virtues and the "sins" to watch out for so you do not become the victim or the cause of harm.

Sex presents many choices. A biological instinct or drive, it can be strong or weak, depending on the person, the circumstances, the timing. Sex can aim toward reproduction or not. Most people want to make love much more often than they want to make babies.

Unlike love, which everyone needs from birth, the sex we are talking about arrives with physical maturity, at adolescence. But readiness for sex takes longer: Emotional maturity and judgment develop more slowly. Unlike love, sex can and should be prepared for. Sex involves passion, and good sex requires control. Sex can intensify love or spoil it.

We look at issues in relationships, not just sex, in this chapter.

These issues are part of intimate, personal, emotional life between two people. Understanding them, being prepared for them, is part of building and maintaining the healthy close relationship that is necessary (but not sufficient) for sex to take place. Learning the difference between infatuation and love, between impulse and commitment, and learning to balance giving and taking, listening and talking — these are some of the things not often taught in class or in books, but they cannot be learned too soon or too well.

Our seven sins against intimacy are violence, cruelty, trespass, infidelity, nagging, contempt and indifference. These sins we talk about are not committed out of meanness, but because people are "stuck" in patterns of behavior — reactions that are hard to control, or habits that are hard to break. It is difficult to change patterns, especially if they have seemed to work in the past, and if they are rooted in strong emotion.

A twosome is the smallest society, and at its best it comes close to heaven on earth. Manners and mores govern the way we act in our closest relationships and with strangers, with friends and with the rest of humanity. Manners and mores are customs or habits that we learn and that gradually change. According to Edmund Burke, in 1797:

> **Manners are of more importance than laws. Upon them, in a great measure, the laws depend. The law touches us but here and there, and now and then. Manners are what vex or smooth, corrupt or purify, exalt or debase, barbarize or refine us, by a constant, steady, uniform, insensible operation, like that of the air we breathe in.**

Seven Sins

To make complicated things simpler, we call good habits virtues, and bad ones sins. Our list of seven sins covers negative behavior quite well, and knowing what *not* to do is the beginning of wisdom and a sign of maturity. Of course, no short list of virtues will cover all good habits, and these have so many different expressions that each person, each couple, can and will develop their own ways of expressing love.

That is why we don't presume to tell you how to be good friends and lovers, yet we think we can help you avoid mistakes that can ruin relationships. Just as it's easier to prevent illnesses than to treat them, so is it easier to prevent relationship problems — which are often bad habits — than to undo them. Just as health is more than the absence of illness, a good relationship involves more than avoiding sin. At the end of the chapter we add a list of virtues, mostly to encourage you to make your own list, your own positive choices. But you must always guard against the pitfalls, since many virtues can be undone by a few sins.

VIOLENCE

There may be reasons for violence, but there are no excuses. If you hit or threaten to hit, you violate the relationship. If you have been hit or threatened with violence, you may choose to give the offender one more chance, but if it happens a second time, you are in an abusive relationship and both of you need help.

Research over the last 20 years shows that leaving a violent relationship (an important option) can be very difficult for some people. The vast majority of victims are female (wives and girlfriends). Usually weaker physically, they are often intimidated by threats of worse violence if they call the police or try to leave. When violence and threats keep someone in a relationship, the result is psychological slavery, or a kind of prison.

Many people wonder how it is possible to love someone who is violent or abusive. For one thing, abuse is often intermittent, not continuous. Abusers may be fine partners much of the time. Many alcoholics, for example, are abusive only when drunk. The victim may have such low self-esteem that she (or he) feels responsible for being hit, for provoking the attack. But no provocation excuses abuse.

Those who live with a violent partner or parent have to deal with love and hate, fear and shame, all mixed together. The mental consequences are often as bad or worse than the physical ones. It's also bad for the mental health of the abuser — violence does not "let off steam," but it does lead to more anger, mixed with guilt, embarrassment, and loss of self-respect.

Physical and psychological abuse tend to go together. Hitting, threatening, insults and name-calling all wreck healthy closeness.

Unfortunately, they may seem "normal" to people who grew up in families where love and good times were mixed with violence and terror. Until recently, police and the courts did not pay much attention to domestic violence. That is now changing with the recognition that most murders occur between acquaintances, including family members, and most assault and battery is domestic violence.

You can be angry. You can argue. You can leave. You can protest with dignity in various ways. But you *must not use or yield to abuse*, verbal or physical. If you are in an abusive relationship or know someone who is, help is available through mental health agencies, legal aid, or child protective services.

The vast majority of Americans do not live in abusive or violent homes, but still encounter violent images and messages all the time, in news and entertainment. Our society is saturated with images and reports of violence, but too little is said and taught about nonviolence.

Nonviolence is not just the absence of hitting. Being nonviolent means that you commit yourself to resolve differences without resorting to violence, verbal or physical. For more guidance on nonviolence, study the ideas of Jesus, Gandhi, Thoreau, Dorothy Day and Martin Luther King.

CRUELTY

Intentionally causing mental pain is what we mean by cruelty. The example we use is a common one: cruel teasing. The better you know someone, the better you know their vulnerabilities, how to hurt their feelings by your actions or with a cutting remark. While a little teasing is normal and fun, there is a point after which it hurts. A loving partner, a good friend, knows that point and will not go past it.

Strong feelings often signal great sensitivity. Feelings (emotions, not thoughts or opinions) create the best and the worst experiences of our lives. Often irrational, feelings are never "ridiculous." The ability to share emotions without fear of humiliation or backlash is the sign of a secure, intimate relationship. If one party turns cruel, and the other tolerates it, the relationship is in trouble.

Why would a friend or lover be cruel? Hurt feelings under the surface sometimes build up. Anger, jealousy, or anxiety may lead to lashing out, which is a clue to something uncomfortable that lies hidden, too deep to recognize.

Boys and girls at puberty are targets for teasing if they develop faster or slower than average, if they are much bigger or smaller than their peers, if they get embarrassed or confused, or if they say too much or too little. Banter and joking arc fun, but everyone knows that hurt feelings result when someone goes too far. If someone does it to you repeatedly, either that person is pushing away from intimacy, or is trying to take over the relationship—dominating instead of sharing.

What should you do in that case, when the teasing has gone too far? If your tormentor says you are too sensitive (a common defense), remind him or her that no one can tell another person how to feel, that sensitivity is a two-way street. The worst thing an offender can say after hurting your feelings is, "Lighten up! Can't you take a joke?" That adds insult to injury.

Contempt

Contempt is anger mixed with disrespect, and it is poisonous. Anger is a normal and often legitimate feeling. It means something needs to be addressed, not that you are free to yell and curse. Friends and lovers must confront problems before anger turns poisonous. John Gottman, a leading researcher on marriage, finds that contempt is associated with a high probability of divorce.

Contempt arises when people are angry and discouraged. It is also a sign of taking someone for granted. It signals that someone is disappointed but, instead of trying to change things for the better, he or she gives up and takes the role of a sore loser. If you think relationships should be easy or should always go your way, you'll be disappointed. If you expect too much or too little, you are likely to be discouraged.

How much can you realistically expect from another person? *You can expect—and you deserve—loving attention to you and the relationship as long as you do the same.* The responsibility for the good and the bad in a relationship is equal until proved otherwise. When things go wrong, you are guilty of contempt if you think either of the following: that it's your partner's fault, or that there's no hope of changing the situation.

Good relationships require some effort, which we think of as "preventive maintenance" rather than work. Romance and courtship are so exciting that everything seems effortless. You're always thinking of, and wanting to please, your partner. After you settle down, things that used to take care of themselves will require some thought.

In real life, routine tends to take over, but that's no sin. It's comforting because it makes life stable and predictable; it's a damper and a disappointment only if there is too little excitement, too little appreciation, or too much taking-for-granted.

If you expect your partner to sparkle all the time, to be available for sex whenever you want it, or to make you feel good all the time, you are expecting too much. The pledge contained in wedding vows reminds us that "for richer and poorer, in sickness and in health, for better and for worse" we will stick together. That commitment, honored over the years, is the difference between love and infatuation.

Besides anger and disrespect, contempt usually involves miscommunication. Let's take some examples.

Miscommunication (failing to make clear what you think and feel): Steve is used to having long conversations on the phone every night with Ellen. He's upset because lately she wants to get off the phone sooner to study, or call a girlfriend. He doesn't talk about it or tell her how he feels, but decides he won't go to the library with her as much. Ellen is upset when he makes excuses to avoid going. They both notice anger and irritability increasing between them, but they don't confront it: Steve never mentioned his hurt feelings directly, and Ellen said nothing about hers.

If you are used to a certain pattern, a change may surprise and upset you. Hurt feelings lead to anger: *Talk about the hurt before anger takes over.* Failing to do so leads to miscommunication. While loving feelings are still strong, say something about the problem *without accusing the other person.*

Steve might have begun: "I didn't realize right away how much it hurt my feelings..." That statement has no anger, no accusatory tone. Instead, when Steve finally admitted his pain, he said, "If you really loved me, you wouldn't cut off the phone calls." Ellen rightly felt that as an attack, and said, "If you really loved me you'd understand—I have other friends, and I have to study." The result is a standoff in which both are disgusted.

Communicate something neutral about your pain before blaming.

Find out whether your partner realizes that you are hurting. Give your partner credit for caring, and talk about the problem. Love means giving the benefit of the doubt: Assume that the other person cares until proved otherwise.

If your partner is withdrawn or angry, it is probably because he or she feels hurt. Instead of accusing, or hoping it will blow over, *take the initiative* and find out what's going on.

Disrespect (you "second guess" instead of taking your partner's word at face value): Angela wears a sexy dress for a big date with Bill, a guy she really likes. Late in the evening, after making out, she says, "I don't want to," when he tries to go all the way. Bill says, "Sure you do!" He wants her to, of course, and hopes she wants to as well. He's partly right, because she may have some mixed feelings (ambivalence). But a "no" has to be respected even when there's some ambivalence. Second-guessing is disrespectful, like saying, "I know your mind better than you do."

Anger or blaming (you make your partner responsible for your own thoughts and feelings): Bill assumes that Angela knows how sexy she is, that she wants him to be aroused, and that she understands how their petting makes him feel. Actions, he figures, speak louder than words: the actions say "yes" even though the words do not. Ignoring what she says, he puts the responsibility (blame) on her for his sexual feelings. Now he wants her to accept the consequences and have intercourse.

Angela is doing some blaming, too. Until now Bill always treated her very well and made her feel wanted, not just for sex but for a serious relationship. She has never felt so loved, and has never been so attracted to anyone. She figures that Bill knew how much she liked him, and is therefore responsible for making her fall in love. But Angela isn't ready for intercourse and has enough doubt to say "stop."

Because Angela says she loves him, Bill cannot understand why she won't have sex with him. Because Bill says he loves her, Angela cannot understand why he won't make a more serious commitment first, like asking her to go with him. The pressure from Bill to have sex equals the pressure from Angela to have a commitment.

But he is 18 and she is 16, and the pressure is too much for them. Bill starts feeling trapped and says Angela is too possessive. As Bill pulls back, Angela feels abandoned and sees him as insincere and over-sexed. Both are angry and blaming. It was her wishful thinking that

Bill wanted commitment, just as it was his wishful thinking that Angela was ready for sex.

In this relationship, each person expected too much, failed to communicate well and started blaming, and now both are stuck with feelings of contempt. He's a lecher, she's a tease.

This is a messy, difficult situation. It's also a very common one, and not just among young people. To protect an intimate relationship you need to pay attention to your partner at the moment you feel most vulnerable. That takes maturity and patience, especially when both of you feel awful and the relationship is "running on empty."

TRESPASS

Crossing a personal limit without permission is trespass. Borrowing someone's things without asking, prying with questions into private matters, reading someone's diary or mail without permission, eavesdropping, and unwelcome touching all violate personal boundaries. In friendship and love we open boundaries willingly, *not under pressure*. This is obviously important when it comes to sex.

Young people often feel that they should not keep anything secret from a best friend, and vice versa. But, as psychologist Erik Erikson taught, real intimacy is possible only after your identity and integrity are ready. Identity means knowing who you are and feeling responsible for yourself. Integrity means being able to defend and assert your identity nonviolently, that is, with respect for the right of others to assert theirs. Adult intimacy means personal sharing by mutual consent. *Intimacy occurs by invitation, by consent, but not by right.*

To put it another way, you have a right *not* to be intimate, but there is no right *to* be intimate. Sexual feelings are strong, and often lead to possessiveness. The personal boundaries of young adults may be insecure, easily violated. If one asks for space, the other *must* back off. To insist on being close against the wishes of another is trespass, which causes pain, fear, embarrassment and anger.

Date rape is an extreme instance of such trespass, even when no violence is involved. An insecure girl may yield to a dominating partner, often an older guy. There may be intimidation or blaming: "You really wanted this or you wouldn't have let me go this far." Alcohol may dull the judgment of one or both. In such cases, sex lacks mutual consent. Recent media coverage and open discussion have increased awareness of this type of violation, but it still occurs too often.

Girls and women are not the only victims of trespass. Boys and men can be and are seduced, harassed, intruded upon. Males, like females, can be hurt by a former (or current) sexual partner. Exposing private information without consent of the other is a form of trespass. It happens to males and females, friends and lovers. It may not be intended to hurt, but it is still the "sin" of trespass.

INFIDELITY

And so we come to the fifth sin, which many people think of first in regard to sex. Infidelity refers to the betrayal of one partner by the other, the destruction of trust. "Infidelity" comes from the Latin *fides*, or trust, and means "not faithful." Take the last example of trespass, having one's secrets exposed: It may or may not be cruel, but it hurts because it is a breach of trust. If you are aware of what hurts a relationship, you will build trust by avoiding those things.

Part of growing up is learning to judge character, which means you become better able to tell who can be trusted. Keeping secrets is a common test among young people. Learning who cannot do that is always a painful experience. Imagine, then, how painful it is to share yourself, *body and soul*, with a partner who betrays you, who becomes unfaithful.

Keeping one's word is another aspect of keeping trust. Promises are made, then kept or broken. There are many small ones, a few large ones, but all promises are important in building trust. "I'll call you tonight." "Let me borrow your pen [notebook, a dollar, etc.] I'll give it back right after school." "I'll be there at seven." Nobody's perfect, but some earn a reputation for being trustworthy. They mean what they say and say what they mean.

Trust builds slowly over time, but it can collapse in a flash. People who care about trust, who speak carefully and keep their word, tend to be equally careful about both large and small things. You can't make up for five broken promises by keeping one big one. There are only so many excuses. For example, being caught in traffic happens. But being late *often* is more than a traffic problem: It's a problem of reliability, thoughtfulness, and trust. Promptness builds trust, tardiness harms it. (If you want to have a later curfew, the way to show your maturity is by keeping the present one faithfully, not by rebelling against it.)

Whole books have been written on fidelity and monogamy (commitment to one partner). Sex symbolizes what is special about marriage and other intimate relationships. Most other things we do with a chosen partner can be done with someone else, but not sex. Infidelity in marriage is called adultery, which has nothing to do with adulthood, but with impurity. "Thou shalt not commit adultery" is the seventh of the Ten Commandments.

Is this rule reasonable and sensible? Take a poll among your friends. If you are in a sexual relationship, do you want your partner to sleep with other people? Chances are you don't. You might discover a double standard; that is, some people feel it is worse for a woman than for a man to be unfaithful. This sexist bias has a long history and is hard — but important — to get rid of.

In our opinion, true intimacy requires fidelity. People do break rules, and the extra attraction of forbidden fruit has a long history. But the costs of lying — guilt, embarrassment and jeopardizing trust — can be huge. Breakers of this rule usually learn the hard way that the pain of infidelity outweighs the pleasure. The Seventh Commandment wasn't written just to keep lechers from having fun, but to warn everyone of the pain of ruined relationships.

NAGGING

After violence, cruelty, contempt, trespass and infidelity, we come to a common sin that is "mortal" only because it is committed so often. Nagging may seem trivial compared with other things, but like little drops of poison it can add up to a lethal dose. We define nagging as asking for the same thing more than twice. That makes almost everyone a nag! Of course, we're concerned about people who do it a lot, without taking responsibility for their part of the problem.

Repeating a request over and over means that either you're asking the wrong person, asking for the wrong thing, or asking in the wrong way. You get frustrated and your partner gets annoyed. "But," you might say, "finally I get results — at least some of the time. If I didn't keep it up, nothing would happen."

Maybe so, but you are describing a poor relationship. When your first two requests are ignored, anger or whining starts: "Why do I always have to ask you ten times?" That's a bad habit that can kill a relationship. You get tired and your partner gets tired. No one causes another person to be a nag. Nagging is the responsibility of the one who keeps asking, and is a sign of low self-esteem and a poor imagination.

Nagging about sex is a drag since sex is supposed to be exciting, romantic, and mutual. But people's needs aren't exactly the same, so a balance or compromise has to be found. When John nags Jane for sex she feels pressure and anxiety, not romance and excitement. When she says "no" he feels rejected, unloved, and weak. She has the power to deny him what he wants. Now sex is at the center of a power struggle. "If you love me you will!" versus "If you love me you won't pressure me." It can get nasty: "If I can't get it from you, I know someone else who wants me!" (That takes us back to infidelity and cruelty.)

Girls nag about sex, too. Guys can withhold it. When that happens, since it is contrary to expectations, it can raise a girl's anxiety about her attractiveness. If she acts desperate, the fun and romance are gone and she makes herself less attractive to him. She may question his manhood, setting him up to prove it, which leads to anxiety, resentment, failure and a dead romance.

Finding a balance takes patience, caring and love. The way two people adjust their sex life reflects how they reach agreement about many things: which television program to watch, which movie or restaurant or concert to go to, which friends to see. Taking turns, being a good sport, paying attention to someone when you would rather be doing something else, playing fair: These things are elementary good manners that should be learned long before sexual feelings come into the picture.

Some people get through childhood without learning how to negotiate with respect. If you're always asking for things more than twice, it's time to talk with your partner about this problem. Say what you mean, and mean what you say. If that doesn't work, it's time to move on — not to the next request but to the next relationship.

INDIFFERENCE

A person may avoid the sins of violence, cruelty, contempt, trespass, infidelity, and nagging. Yet by *not caring*, that person can still destroy the relationship. In a way, indifference is the opposite of nagging—the other extreme. Instead of pestering, the person withdraws. Notice that we have not included hatred as a sin, though it can destroy a relationship; but hate is a sign of powerful emotion, as is love, while indifference is the opposite of both. It is an absence of emotion. Indifference toward people we hardly know is understandable, but to know someone well and be uncaring really hurts.

As we have pointed out, teasing your partner by doing (or saying) things you know are hurtful is cruel. Here we consider the consequence of not noticing, not caring. Indifference may be passive (not intentional) but it can hurt as much as cruelty.

If you know what your partner likes, wants, and hates, you will, to keep up a good relationship, show that you care about those things, too. That doesn't mean you have to feel the same way he or she does about everything. It means that you pay respectful attention to preferences that may *not* be yours; we assume your partner will do the same. That's what love is all about.

For example, if you hate each other's favorite music, you will still buy a recording that your partner likes for a birthday gift. You don't have to listen to it, although that would be a nice gesture if you can refrain from snide remarks! When you are in the car together, you will find a compromise when listening to the radio. Taking turns, perhaps, or finding some middle ground, avoiding what annoys either one of you.

Unless we meet the most important needs of a loved one, the relationship will die. This is especially true for those needs that we alone can satisfy, or for the needs we create—for companionship, support, and sex.

Jane needs Joe and he says he's busy watching a game on TV. She's hurt. Another time, Joe needs Jane and she wants to go to the mall with a girlfriend. He's hurt. Neither wants to hurt the other. Either might say, "I made plans to do this a long time ago," or, "I just needed some space." But one party feels the other is indifferent and the relationship starts to turn sour.

The hurt was done unintentionally, so the offender is often puzzled and defensive. "I didn't mean to hurt you" is a true and appropriate statement. "You're just too sensitive" is a judgment to be avoided. It just adds insult to injury.

It takes maturity, experience, flexibility and sensitivity to diagnose indifference when people are fighting about it. Teenagers spend a lot of time thinking and talking about relationships in addition to complaining: "He doesn't care enough!"; "She's too sensitive!"; and vice versa.

Empathy is knowing and caring about what another person feels. Routine without empathy is deadly because each partner seems indifferent to the other's emotion or state of mind. In real love empathy becomes a habit, part of the routine that keeps romance alive. Then you have something wonderful, a relationship greater than the sum of its parts.

Seven Virtues

Although we have been addressing problems and their prevention, we are optimists about teens and their ability to cope with relationship changes. As we said, many virtues can be undone by a few sins. By avoiding these pitfalls, you have many choices, better teamwork, and more happiness. Like a travel guide, this book warns you about dangers while preparing you for a wonderful experience. By preparing, you will have a much better time. Part of the adventure is finding things you didn't expect. Even the best guidebook cannot predict what you will enjoy most, only that the trip will be worthwhile, you will learn, have fun, encounter and resolve problems, find new friends and new interests — maybe love.

To address virtues, to develop choices, to decide who you want to be and who you want to be with, takes time, experience, reflection, and guidance. As a start then, not as a final list, we offer seven virtues, like a guidebook telling just a few things that must not be missed on your journey. Virtues are harder to define and have many manifestations. They keep relationships strong and satisfying. These virtues are *nonviolence, kindness, humor, respect, fidelity, listening* and *caring*. Develop these, and make your own list. Discuss these ideas, both the negative and positive sides. Your ideas will change with experience and understanding.

Identify your values and you forge an identity.

Chapter 2

Abstinence

The capacity for sustained abstinence precedes the capacity for a genuine choice. —Anna Freud

Whether or not you have ever had sexual experience with a partner you can practice abstinence: You can choose not to have sex. You cannot become a virgin again, but you can change from active to abstinent. Many people do this voluntarily; everyone does it at times out of necessity. Illness, injury, distance from one's partner, and relationship problems all interrupt a sexual relationship.

Here we will emphasize the decision to have sex for the first time, providing reasons both for and against that decision. We strongly believe that sex should only be part of a good, stable, loving relationship, an ideal that is not always met in real life. A great deal of pain occurs in the lives of women and men, young and old, because that ideal is not observed. Seeking pleasure at the expense of another, or using sex to control or influence a relationship selfishly, is a recipe for disaster.

Most religions have rules about sex — requiring abstinence until marriage, for example. The observant may not have an easy time following the rule, but many do; those who do not, often feel guilty. People who seem to lack a clear set of rules about sexual intercourse still abstain for various reasons. Abstaining for personal health and well-being (avoiding the risk of pregnancy and disease) is simple common sense. Abstaining for the sake of the relationship (when one partner — or perhaps both — does not feel ready) is sensible, if not simple, and involves some consideration for the partner. Sometimes people abstain without knowing why: it just feels right. The reasons for abstinence are complex, perhaps more so than the reasons for having sex.

Abstinence usually means refraining from sexual intercourse. Of course, people also abstain from other forms of sexual activity. Some religions forbid or discourage masturbation, sexual thoughts, or homosexuality. Some people are uncomfortable with certain sexual practices like oral or anal sex and abstain from them, even though someone else — perhaps their partners — consider them "exciting." Abstinence is practiced by teens and adults, virgins and nonvirgins, for various lengths of time and for various reasons.

Reasons for Abstaining

Why do many teens decide to abstain from having sex? For starters, it is 100 percent effective in preventing pregnancy and STDs. But reasons range from "It is my personal decision to remain chaste for Jesus" to "I couldn't find anyone to do it with me if I tried," and many reasons in between. A few personal stories might seem familiar:

> Stephanie's reason for "no sex now" is a result of mature thinking on her part. At 17, she is sure that having sex with any of the boys she dates would create serious problems for her. "When a boy I like even touches me, I practically fall in love with him," she explains, "and then I become too involved and too possessive. What would happen if I went all the way instead of just part way? I'd make a fool of myself. I'd be so emotional about him and so preoccupied — thinking and worrying about him all the time — that it would drive me, and probably the guy, crazy. I might have sex with a boy before marriage. I don't have any moral hang-ups, just emotional ones; but that's enough reason to wait."
>
> * * *
>
> Josh, 18, is popular, a good athlete, and a leader in his church youth group. "Look," he says, "my mom had me when she was 16. She had a rough time, having to work, raising me by herself until my stepdad came into the picture when I was seven. We have a good family now. Sure, I could have sex, but I know that any girl I'd be interested in would want more than a roll

in the hay. So would I. If it was just playing around with someone I didn't care about it wouldn't be right. I know a lot of guys whose lives got messed up that way, along with their girlfriends': Even if they don't get pregnant, the girls feel used."

Research

Although more teens are having sex before marriage than in past generations, they do not begin as early as many people think. It may surprise most Americans to know that over half of teenagers are virgins at least until 17. And while the incidence of intercourse increases with age, 20 percent abstain throughout their teen years. Those concerned with *premarital* sex must remember that the average age of marriage has risen about four years since 1950. In the fifties, women often married right out of high school — half of those who would ever marry were brides by the time they were 20. Now half are still single at 24, and there are far fewer teen brides. For males, the average age at marriage used to be 23; now it is 26.

Research also shows that teens who engage in other high risk behavior — smoking, drinking, and drug use — are most likely to have sex early. Even those who have become sexually active can and do become abstainers again, as we have mentioned. About a third of non-virgin women had not had sex in the month before a survey; one-quarter had sex in fewer than six months out of a year after they first experienced intercourse.

Although she is not a virgin, Eileen, almost 18, practices abstinence. Two years ago she had a sexual experience that turned out badly. "The guy used me. He just wanted to have sex — he didn't care about me. I'm not turned off to guys or anything like that," she explained. "But at this point I really think of myself as a virgin again. I don't count that 'first time' at all. That was not what sex is supposed to be. I regret it, but it will make me be a lot more careful next time. Meanwhile I've seen too many girlfriends get pregnant, have abortions or drop out to raise a kid without the father — these guys aren't about to take the responsibility!"

* * *

Laurie, who is 16, comes from a conservative background. Her parents don't shield her from exposure to sex in the media — she can watch TV and see movies with her friends — but they have made clear to her through words and their own lifestyle their strong beliefs about love and sex: Wait until marriage for sex. Her mother did not sleep with Laurie's father prior to marriage, and says she feels very good about this choice. Laurie's parents seem very happy. There are lots of people who "preach" to teenagers, but her parents practice what they preach. Laurie has always been treated with respect and love by her parents, and she is impressed by the moral stand they take and respects them for it — so her commitment to chastity is strong, based on positive identification, not fear and shame.

* * *

Paul is 17. He explains, "When I was 16 I had relations with a girl who was also 16. Neither of us knew what we were doing. We were not 'in love' enough to be very romantic. It happened in a car, and it was really awkward. When it was over I couldn't think of anything to say. It was really quiet and weird. The next day I got worried she might be pregnant. I tried to learn all I could about whether I might become a father at 17! I did a lot of reading and learned a lot more about sex. I also learned that there's a lot more to having sex than I thought there was — physically and emotionally. I'm not ready for sex and I don't think any girl my age is either."

* * *

Stacy, 15, has been dating Jake, 16, for about 6 months. He has had sexual intercourse before, but she has not. They have been talking about it a lot recently because Jake feels ready. Stacy would like to try it — she loves Jake and thinks he would be a very caring and romantic "first love." But she is too scared to go all the way. "I've heard a lot about people doing it even once and getting pregnant or getting AIDS and I just don't feel like risking that. I know that we can get condoms or the pill, but those things aren't 100 percent perfect. Sometimes I imagine what it would feel like waking up one morning and finding out

I was pregnant or that Jake or I had AIDS and I just get this sick feeling in my stomach. I couldn't deal; I think I would worry about it even while we were having sex so I couldn't really relax and enjoy it. I know people who've done it and don't seem to worry, but I also know some who have done it and regret it. Why rush something that's supposed to be wonderful if you can ruin it that way?"

* * *

George, now 19, explains his past experiences. "I had gone steady with Paula for over two years. Twice during our relationship we were very close to going all the way. We were in love with each other and were planning marriage in the future, but for some reason we didn't go all the way. She put the brakes on both times. Now I find I don't love her any more and I want to break up with her. Had we gone all the way last year, we might have had to get married, either because she got pregnant, or because we felt emotionally obligated. If that had happened we'd be miserable together, or divorced."

There are plenty of guys who will sleep with an "easy mark" for fun but want to marry a virgin. This is an example of what is called the double standard: boys who believe it's all right for them to have sex before marriage, but not for the "nice" marrying girls. Some women play this game, too: They think it's important to be a virgin themselves, but it's okay, even better, if the bridegroom has had some experience.

This double standard, or hypocrisy, can lead to real problems. For the guy there may be two categories of female: the sexually free one, and the proper wife-and-mother type. Impotence or lack of sexual interest becomes a problem in long-term relationships — including marriage — for some of these men because they can't relate to a woman who is both sexual and a "good woman." For women, too, there can be a psychological split between sex-for-kicks and loving sex. The best sex occurs when fun and the loving are integrated. Think about it. If good looks and sex appeal were the keys to successful relationships, there would be no divorces among Hollywood stars. People who realize that there is so much more involved, and that true intimacy is worth waiting for, confidently choose abstinence.

Paul, Josh and George show the extent to which boys choose abstinence for the short or long term. Laurie's conservative position deserves respect, as does Stephanie's need to maintain a measure of emotional independence. Although Eileen was hurt by one bad experience, she shows a healthy reluctance to repeat that experience, not an extreme fear of sex or men in general. Stacy's concerns about pregnancy and HIV/AIDS show her to be mature and sensible. Having sex always brings with it some level of risk, even when partners take precautions, and that must always be factored into the equation.

Which of the above teenagers should be concerned about contraception now? *All of them.* Even if moral principles do not change, Laurie should be aware that perspectives do change with experience; and, so far, her emotions have not been seriously tested. What if Stephanie finds the emotional security she needs as a prerequisite to sex? What if Eileen's next boyfriend invites sex as part of love, not exploitation? And what if Stacy decides that she's ready for sex, as long as it's safe? As for Josh, Paul and George, like the girls, they need to know about contraception in case the right relationship comes along, even if they plan to wait until marriage. All of these thoughtful young people may be in a position to advise and influence friends — yet another reason to be well informed. There is a lot of misinformation out there!

Any or all of these young people may soon find themselves seriously involved and on the verge of having sex. Unfortunately, the excitement of love or passion often interferes with taking the time to get one's facts straight about pregnancy, sexually transmitted diseases and contraception. Being abstinent doesn't mean you aren't thinking about sex somewhere down the road. In fact, it can be a very good time to gradually gather information about birth control so that you understand your options when the time comes, even if it's years away. Kids can be "in the know" without having early sexual experience. In fact, often times those who boast of sexual experience are the most insecure and misinformed.

Reasons for Not Abstaining

If there is a common feeling underlying what was said by all these teenagers, it can be summed up in three words: "I'm not ready." For them — and for you if you have similar feelings — sexual abstinence makes sense. Abstaining from sex has a value, and that value is far greater than biological safety or protection against criticism. It has to do with a sense of readiness, a wish to make sex both a physically and emotionally special experience when the person, time, and place are right.

"Readiness" is a useful concept in human development. Take, for example, "reading readiness." Your vision, ability to concentrate, and other brain functions must be at a certain level before you can learn to read. Readiness means you have potential to be competent, to learn skills or concepts which were beyond your capacity before. The nerves and muscles must be formed and teachable, the mind must be ready to acquire and digest new information, and the emotions must be in harmony with the task ahead.

With sex, physical readiness develops before emotional readiness. Those who do not wait for emotional readiness are usually disappointed by sex, and many are harmed by it. It is impossible to explain emotional readiness, or maturity, to someone who isn't there yet. You can talk about it, but it won't mean much — like describing what it's like to speak a second language to someone who has never done it. And people become ready in different ways, at different times, and all go through anxiety and doubt in the process.

One factor that complicates the issue of being "ready" for sex is physical readiness. Over the years, average age at first menstruation has been slowly going down, probably because of better nutrition, and is now 12.5 years of age. Meanwhile, the median age at first marriage has been rising and is now the highest it has ever been: 24 for women and 26 for men. That means that young people are becoming fertile earlier and are getting married much later, which has led to much longer periods of time during which they are physically capable of sex and childbearing but are unmarried. How do you handle that decade or so?

Asking the Right Questions

Here are a few ideas and cases that can help you form guidelines for yourself as you decide between abstinence and sex.

Can the two of you discuss birth control?

Working out the details of contraception should be shared by a couple. It reflects maturity and shows you care about each other, yourself, the people around you, and the society you live in.

> Estelle does not know how to bring up the subject with her boyfriend. "I'd be too embarrassed — what could I say? I know he wants to have sex, and I wish he would talk about birth control, because he makes me feel that I'm not romantic and I don't love him because I'm worried about the logistics of sex when all he talks about is the intimacy of it. I feel guilty that I'm holding back."

How about asking one question: "If we have sex, what will we use for protection?" If you are too shy to ask, you are certainly not ready for sex. If your boyfriend (or girlfriend) can't give a straight and serious answer, he or she is not ready either. Two people who can't wait to have sex but who are too embarrassed to talk about birth control are like people who love whitewater rafting but are embarrassed to admit they'd feel safer wearing lifejackets. Estelle may be afraid to find out that her boyfriend doesn't care enough about her to bother with protection: Some guys don't want to admit that there's any risk at all. On the flip side, his agreement to get and use contraception may not, by itself, make you feel ready, and that's okay, too. Emotional and social readiness are entirely separate from "contraceptively ready." This much is certain: If you can't talk about protection and do something about it, you are not ready for sex.

Girls: Will having sex make him call more, care more?
Guys: Will having sex mean that she's your girl?
Are you hoping that sex will improve your relationship? Don't count on it. It's as likely to hinder as it is to help. As the involvement gets deeper, the risks are greater and the stakes are higher. You've probably seen lots of relationships crash and burn. Premature sex can be one cause.

> Leonard, 18, tells it this way: "I think Mary was using sex to try and keep me dating her. When we started dating, she would barely let me touch her, but when I started getting interested in another girl, suddenly Mary's 'no' turned to 'go.' We were

watching TV in her basement and she whispered to me to undo her bra. That got to me. I kept thinking what a mess it would be if she got pregnant, with me not even liking her any more. We did it, and I stopped seeing her after that night."

That's desperation sex. Many teenagers learn this lesson the hard way. If the relationship isn't good, consummating it sexually can't improve it. Instead, the poor relationship will drag the sex down to its level.

Do you have any guilty feelings about how far you've gone already?

Guilt takes many forms. "I went too far" is one sign. Sheila looks forward to petting to climax with her boyfriend, but afterwards wonders if what they are doing is "moral" or right. Her guilt shows itself in her being irritable on mornings following her dates. She is unhappy with herself and embarrassed around her family. She tries to push back her guilt by being scrupulously "good," but then she "snaps" with anger, sometimes at her mother, sometimes at her boyfriend. Sometimes she will "punish" herself after a date by staying up and studying a couple of hours until she is totally exhausted. She seems to be unconsciously making a bargain: "If I get good grades, that will pay for my bad morals."

Sex is not a slippery slope. Just because you've engaged in petting with your partner or had oral sex doesn't mean you must go on to the "next base." If you feel any guilt, doubt, or conflict about going as far as you already have gone, then you are not ready to go further. You may even feel better taking a step back.

Are you thinking about sex all the time, wanting to have sex just to "get it out of your system"?

Boys, especially, have strong sexual urges and frequent sexual daydreams. Having sex just to get it out of your system doesn't work. If it's good you'll want more, if it's not you'll want to try again, and if it's terrible you'll be sorry you did it. Experimenting out of curiosity or desperation usually leads to disappointment or failure. If you're obsessed with sexual thoughts now, imagine how it will be when another person is involved. You'll not only have the thoughts, but you'll have the added worries about your feelings for the other person, her feelings for you, and any physical consequences (pregnancy or disease) that could occur. If masturbation doesn't control sexual urges, why should intercourse? If masturbation causes guilt, or if pressure to have intercourse interferes with normal friendships and social activities, then the need for professional help is indicated.

> David was obsessed with sex, and couldn't get his mind off a particular girl in his class. He felt he didn't have a chance with her, and his infatuation turned to resentment. He made an obscene phone call, saying he wanted to screw her; then another and another. Finally she recognized his voice and he is now getting the psychiatric help he needs.

This is just one example of how immature sexual behavior changes good feelings into bad experience.

Are you jealous of the person you're dating, and do you believe that having sex with him or her will change that?
A little jealousy is okay — it's flattering to the partner. But too much makes a person feel like a captive instead of a willing partner in a relationship, which can be disastrous. Excessive fear of loss or betrayal can be a "self-fulfilling prophecy." Constant questions, suspicion, and possessiveness can put out the spark in any relationship. Having sex only adds fuel to the fire of jealousy because it raises the stakes and can make the jealous person cling even more.
Lisa, 16, provides a typical example. When her boyfriend talks to other girls at parties, she seethes inside. She feels hurt and angry. Conversations such as this follow:

> LISA: Well, you certainly seemed to be having a good time.
> BEN: Yeah, weren't you?
> LISA: Well, I might have had a good time if you hadn't neglected me most of the evening.
> BEN: For heaven's sake, I was just talking to Pat and Linda for a few minutes.
> LISA: Oh, they're more interesting to talk to than I am, I suppose...

That last remark gets at the heart of Lisa's problem. She feels insecure compared to other girls, afraid that she's less interesting. Lacking self-confidence, she is quick to see other girls as competition.

Would it be different if Lisa and Ben were having sex? Yes, the situation would be different — but probably worse for Lisa. She would feel doubly "damaged," hurt and angry. If she is bothered that a boy she dates would talk to other girls, how would she feel if a boy she slept with talked to other girls? Does she — do you? — think adding sex to the mixture would keep Ben from having normal conversation with other girls? Should it? No! Lisa needs to gain confidence in herself before she is ready for sex. She has to stop seeing every girl as competition, and her boyfriend as her possession. Being or having a "one and only" should leave room for friends of the opposite sex. This is as true for couples who are intimate sexually as it is for those who abstain. Though our example here is Lisa, boys are equally prone to jealousy. (Try switching male and female roles in the dialogue.)

What do you imagine as a possible result of a sexual involvement?

Random thoughts, fantasies, or daydreams can provide clues to your underlying motives for wanting sex; they can help tell you whether your motives are healthy or not. Do you envision sudden, dramatic gossip among your friends? ("Guess who's sleeping together?...") If so, you may want sex as an attention-getting technique, and you'd be wise to explore other ways to get the recognition you are seeking.

Do you have thoughts of parental outrage or hand-wringing? ("Where did we go wrong?") If so, then sex for you may be a means of rebellion — not primarily an expression of love. In that case, you may be exploiting your partner in order to provoke your parents.

If you are a male hoping to win your girl's heart by "making the earth move" with your lovemaking, you may be in for disappointment. A good sexual relationship takes time — Hollywood depictions notwithstanding. The male's physical pleasure is almost guaranteed, but the girl's may be somewhat unpredictable. If you allow your ego to rise and fall with her sexual response, she'll feel the pressure and it will hinder, not help, the response you hope for. She might fake it just to please you and get it over with, or she'll resent the pressure and your original goal of getting closer to her will backfire.

Are you trying to prove something by having sex?

Do you imagine sex removing doubts about your attractiveness, your sexiness, your personal worth? You may saddle your sex with a load of worries that it cannot carry. Using sex to solve problems — like building up weak egos — interferes with good sex. Remember, every-one has some insecurities, and being in love with someone means that you trust they will not take advantage of your vulnerabilities. But if you are feeling shaky at the start, sex slides quickly from sham — "I can do this, I've seen it in the movies"— into shame: "Yecch. I can't believe I actually did that with him [her]." Tentative sex is like a shaky bridge: You might get across, but the journey may make you sick and even instill a fear of heights.

Sex can't create the foundation for a good relationship. What it can provide is additional mortar between the bricks — it can solidify and strengthen the partnership when it's already strong. Sex is give-and-take; as in duets, two soloists don't do well, nor do two accompanists. You have to know when to take the lead, when to fade back, and how to blend. It takes practice, patience, skill, trust and love. It also takes confidence. Even the most loving couples may feel awkward or stumble in the beginning. But because they are sensitive to each other's feelings and can communicate about their hopes, disappointments and thoughts about sex, they can make it work. If you're having sex to try and prove something to yourself, or even to someone else, you're not ready for sex.

Are you feeling pressured to have sex?

Pressure for sex is all around us. Everyone seems to be doing it — on television, in movies, among friends — and they all seem to enjoy it. Hardly any regrets, hardly any pregnancies, hardly any mention of birth control. Come on, let's get real! With all that sex and no birth control, there are going to be a lot of unintended pregnancies and a lot of regrets. Passionate sex on the screen sells more household products and cars than, say, a story of disappointing sex or a story about abstinence. But those people in the movies are reading lines from a script, not negoti-ating complex, lasting life decisions.

For boys in general, and insecure girls in particular, it is often eas-ier to say "yes" to sex than "no." But don't be fooled. Having sex because "everyone else is doing it" means you are giving other people's reasons more weight than your own. Any reason for not having sex is a good enough reason, whether clearly thought out or just a "gut feeling." Lots of reasons for having sex are *not* good.

Not feeling ready even if "everyone else" seems to be (they often find out later that they weren't) is hard. A person will sometimes try to make a cautious partner, the "hold out," feel less grown up for not having sex. It's a trick to get what they want, like saying, "If you really loved me, you would." The answer to that is, "If you really loved me, you'd back off!" Friendly persuasion is one thing, but real grownups don't pester, or threaten, to get sex in a loving relationship. If it's not a loving relationship, then sex shouldn't be part of it.

Pressure comes from many sources; the hardest to resist comes from your boyfriend or girlfriend. When one of you is ready to have sex and the other is not, what do you say? Discuss how you feel and try to understand where the other person is coming from. Beware of pressure tactics like "we're going to get married eventually, so why wait?" Some things are worth waiting for, and this is one of them. Taking a line from one sex education campaign: "Abstinence makes the heart grow fonder." The bottom line is that if you're not ready, and your partner is not willing to wait until you are, you are better off without him or her than compromising your principles.

One special circumstance to consider is when a significant age difference exists between partners. A recent study found that almost two-thirds of teen mothers age 15–19 have partners who are 20 or older. One in five teen mothers aged 15–17 have a partner who is six or more years older. The researchers state that "this type of age difference suggests, at the least, very different levels of life experience and power, and brings into question issues of pressure and abuse. Data from the National Survey of Children indicate that about 18 percent of women 17 and younger who have had intercourse were forced at least once to do so" (Landry et al.). That statistic speaks volumes about one kind of pressure to have sex — physical pressure.

Developmentally, age differences become less important as people grow older. Is four years a big difference? Compare a couple consisting of a 16- and a 20-year-old with one consisting of a 36- and 40-year-old. As people age, the gap narrows in terms of life experiences, social development and other factors. A 16-year-old girl is certainly the underdog physically, emotionally and intellectually when it comes to negotiating with a 20-year-old man about sex ... or any other life decisions. In some cases, age-of-consent laws prohibit adolescents and adults from having sex. Even in cases where the relationship is consensual, we strongly recommend reassessing the "wisdom of the relationship." Why would a young girl want to be with someone so much older than herself? Status? A (false) sense of security? What can an adult man get from a teenage girl that he can't find in a woman his own age? Power and authority, if he is insecure. Questions like these may reveal motives that have little to do with love and intimacy and a lot to do with insecurity and power struggles.

The last question to ask yourself before deciding to begin a sexual relationship might be: How much deception will likely result?
Consideration not only for yourself but for your parents, the community in general, and even for your good friends will require that you not broadcast the facts of your affair. On the contrary, discretion or even secrecy might be required.

Discretion about a sexual affair, however, is different from deceit. If a girl tells her parents, "We'll be at Kara's house," when she and her boyfriend are actually going to a friend's apartment, there is always a risk that parents may call Kara's house to "check up." The beauty of sexual intimacy can be easily spoiled by the tension that results from false stories and alibis. You may be ready for a sexual affair, but circumstances won't permit it without deception or outright lies. In that case, patience is in order.

There is a very delicate balance here. Your sex life is private, and you don't have to discuss it with anyone, and probably shouldn't unless you are talking to your lover, doctor, or counselor. This means that there may be times when you do not tell your parents or others the "whole truth and nothing but the truth." But most people find that if they get involved in a web of deceptions and outright lies, the price is high — in terms of guilt that interferes with sexual pleasure, the stress of constantly having to "cover your tracks," and in the loss of trust from friends and family if the truth comes out (it often does).

What About Love?

We have not asked, "Are you in love?" It's often too difficult to know. And when does that make a difference? If sex is okay when you're in love, then it's all too easy to say and believe, "Well, we're in love, so let's have sex." We believe that love is necessary, but not sufficient.

The words "I love you" do not guarantee that the feeling really exists. Love involves not only caring about another person, but also feelings of esteem for yourself. To discover if you really hold those feelings of esteem, it is necessary to ask deeper questions than just "Am I in love?" It is also important to consider issues of mutual respect, trust, and maturity.

Of course love is relevant to sex. If you consider the quality of a sexual experience — Was it all you hoped it would be? Did it bring happiness? — then love becomes extremely important. However you define love, most people feel that without it sex is unsatisfying, empty, cheap, or worse (disgusting). The ideal — and for many people the only situation they really want — is sex with love.

How you decide is as important as *what* you decide. Saying "yes" to sex responsibly is only possible if you are capable of saying "no." If you cannot abstain, you cannot choose — you merely react. Choosing whether or not to have sex requires getting in touch with your mind and your body. If it feels like a huge decision, that's because it is. And not just the "first time" — sex is a big deal every time because it is powerful, intimate, and carries with it inherent risks, both emotional (being vulnerable) and physical (pregnancy and STDs, including HIV/AIDS). Sex and abstinence are both normal, healthy aspects of human relations and they are capable of being used well or badly.

Frequently Asked Questions

Isn't it unhealthy to refrain from sex? After all, you're repressing a natural drive, aren't you?

Sex is not necessary to life in the same way as are eating, sleeping or breathing. Sex is "natural" but not biologically essential. Sexual drives vary from person to person, and from time to time. Furthermore, most teenagers with strong sexual urges find masturbation or petting or erotic dreams to be outlets that decrease tension and help them abstain from premature intercourse.

If you don't have sex in your teens, are you likely to be frigid or impotent when you're an adult?

No. Bad early experience is much more likely to produce problems later on. It depends on readiness, and why you do or don't have sex. Teens who abstain do so for a variety of reasons; these include morality, anxiety or just plain choosiness.

Can you have oral sex and still call it abstinence?

It is not actual intercourse, and pregnancy cannot result. But that is technical abstinence. Oral sex is just as intimate and involving as intercourse. Some teenagers find oral sex fully satisfying; a few, in fact, consider it their means of birth control. Most, however, do not engage in oral sex until after they have had intercourse for some time, and some never do. Some people consider it very advanced, while others consider it a form of mutual masturbation. Some do consider it abstinence, which it is in a narrow sense only.

Do adults practice abstinence?

Of course. Single men and women often abstain from sex when a satisfactory partner is not available. Married couples may abstain when they are in the midst of an argument, when one partner is ill, when the usual method of contraception is not available, when husband or wife is out of town, or for other reasons. And for married Catholic couples who use the rhythm method of birth control, calculated periods of abstinence from intercourse are a must! Such couples could not use oral sex as an alternative because their religion teaches abstinence from all forms of sexual expression except intercourse — and that without artificial contraception. Adults, like teenagers, have religious, emotional, physical and other factors to consider when deciding whether or not to practice abstinence.

Chapter 3

Infection and Disease

A bacillus dividing once every hour would at the end of 24 hours have increased to 17,000,000. ... They are in the air we breathe, the water and milk we drink, upon the exposed surfaces of man and animals, and in their intestinal tracts, and in the soil to a depth of about nine feet. —William Osler, M.D., 1901

There are good germs, bad germs, and neutral germs. They are small, and they are many. As Dr. Osler wrote (before the discovery of viruses, which are 10 to 100 times smaller than bacteria), they are all over us, even inside us in some places. Most are helpful or harmless, breaking down our food, dead cells and other organic matter. Even bad germs, or pathogens, don't always cause trouble: It depends where they attack, how many there are, and what kind of defenses we have. These "bugs" are so small you cannot see them, but there are so many that they amount to ten percent of our body weight and about half the intestinal contents.

Gonococcus, tuberculosis, streptococcus ("strep"), and staphylococcus ("staph") are some bacteria that cause infections; herpes and human immunodeficiency virus (HIV) are harmful viruses that make us ill. This chapter concentrates on diseases spread through sexual contact. Other types of infection can be transmitted through the air by coughing and sneezing, by touch, or by ingesting contaminated food or water.

We have defense systems against infection, and we can assist the body in its efforts to resist such invasions. Cooking food well protects against hepatitis and dysentery. Washing hands before eating and after using the toilet protects against spreading harmful germs from one area to another. Covering mouth and nose when coughing or sneezing protects others from our germs. Using only your own towel, washcloth, toothbrush and comb also protects you from exposure to germs from others.

Some people carry germs that cause them no problem but are harmful to others. These "carriers" may not be aware that they are a source of infection; they may have immunity due to previous exposure. Also, people often spread germs in the first days of their exposure, even before they know they are sick. You, they, even a doctor cannot tell they are contagious. By the same token, people can catch and carry herpes and other sexually transmitted diseases without knowing they've been exposed! Three conditions must exist for infection to occur. First, the germ has to be present. Second, there must be a host, in this case a person, to receive the germ. Third, conditions must favor the germ so that it multiplies.

Working against infection is the body's immune system, particularly white blood cells, which attack the invading germ. The immune system functions best when we get enough rest, proper nutrition, exercise, fresh air, and keep our stress levels from rising too high. AIDS — Acquired Immunodeficiency Syndrome — is so deadly because it destroys the immune system, leaving the infected person more vulnerable to serious diseases than a person with a healthy immune system.

Antibiotics like penicillin have been very effective in combating disease since their introduction in the 1940s, but many germs have grown resistant to them. This is largely because these "wonder drugs" have been prescribed too often.

Some germs — bacteria, viruses, yeasts, protozoa — and some larger invaders like lice are transmitted primarily through sex. The infections, which used to be called venereal diseases (from venery/Venus), now are referred to as sexually transmitted diseases (STDs), sexually transmitted infections or reproductive tract infections (we use STD in this book). The anus, vagina, and penis are moist, warm and dark, a paradise for germs. While anal sex has no pregnancy risk, it exposes those who practice it to bacterial and viral risk; the same is true for oral sex. With vaginal intercourse both risks exist.

Sexually Transmitted Diseases (STDs)

Among teens, which is more common, pregnancy or STDs?

According to the Centers for Disease Control and Prevention, 12 million Americans get an STD annually. In 1995, three of the top ten reported infectious diseases were STDs: chlamydia, gonorrhea and AIDS. *Three million teenagers contract an STD every year.* That's 25 percent of all STD cases, and it is also 25 percent of sexually active teenagers. That means three times as many teenagers are getting STDs as are getting pregnant each year! These germs respect no boundaries of age, gender or race. Anyone exposed to an infected partner is at risk.

Sexually transmitted diseases (STDs) are infections that spread through sexual contact that includes vaginal and anal intercourse and oral sex. More than 20 microbes can be transmitted this way. Some common ones are chlamydia and gonorrhea, caused by bacteria; human immunodeficiency virus (HIV) and herpes, caused by viruses; and trichomoniasis, caused by a protozoan. (Candidiasis, a yeast infection, and bacterial vaginosis are syndromes that are not considered sexually transmitted infections, though they are, in rare instances, transmitted through sexual contact.)

The health consequences of STDs range from mild, temporary problems to serious life-threatening illnesses. Bacterial infections can be cured with medications, but left untreated they can cause problematic pregnancies and infertility. No cure has yet been found for viral diseases, some of which can be prevented with vaccination, but there are some treatments that help control symptoms.

Certain factors place some people at greater risk:

• Most STDs are more easily transmitted to women than to men. For biological reasons, a woman is twice as likely as a man to contact gonorrhea, chlamydia or hepatitis B during unprotected intercourse with an infected partner.

• People who already have an active STD are more likely to contract HIV than other people because it is easier for HIV to enter the body through irritated genital tissue and sores.

• HIV can also be transmitted through anal and oral sex. Using a latex condom during oral and anal sex can help protect against trans-mission. Lesbian couples can use a dental dam during oral sex, a thin square of latex that is placed between the mouth of one partner and the genitals of another.

• Having more than one sex partner increases the risk of exposure. By 12th grade about three-fourths of high school students have had sex-ual intercourse, and about one-fifth have had more than four sex part-ners. This is risky business.

• Physiological factors related to age, such as an immature immune system, increase the likelihood of teens getting STDs from unprotected sex.

• Using a latex condom correctly provides excellent protection against STDs, but only 29 percent of sexually active teens use condoms consistently.

Most people underestimate STDs, not realizing how widespread and dangerous they are. A Gallup poll found that teenagers know more than adults about STDs, but STD knowledge is low overall. For exam-ple, only 12 percent of teens and four percent of adults knew that STDs infect one in five people; 26 percent of adults and 42 percent of teens could not name an STD other than HIV/AIDS. A larger number — 83 percent of teens and 66 percent of adults — knew that some STDs besides HIV/AIDS are incurable.

How can you protect yourself from STDs? Don't have sex with anyone who might be infected. That means either (1) abstain com-pletely, or (2) make sure your partner is uninfected and absolutely faith-ful to you.

The latex condom protects quite well against STDs, including HIV/AIDS, but is not 100 percent effective. So the term "safe sex" is somewhat misleading. Sex isn't risk-free, and "safer sex" better describes sex with the protection of a latex condom. (See Chapter 4 for more information about latex and "skin" condoms and STDs.)

If you choose to have sex, be careful. Take the same precautions with STDs that you would with any threat to your health.

• Learn the best ways to protect yourself from getting the disease — avoid likely sources of infection; don't take chances — as with pregnancy, the moments of pleasure must be balanced with concern for all the con-sequences of sex, physical and emotional;

• Know the symptoms; if you have any, see a health professional;

• If you have possibly been exposed to an STD, don't wait for symptoms. Get tested right away and *don't expose anyone else* until you've been medically cleared;

• If there's a chance you have transmitted an infection, let the other person or persons know about it so they can seek treatment for themselves (in case they have not yet noticed any symptoms). And they should notify anyone else they may have infected. The consequences of sex can be far-reaching.

Learning you have an STD can be a shock, but having it and not knowing it is much worse. Knowing enables you to get treatment and do some thinking.

> In Donna's case, learning was a double shock: she thought she was Jason's one-and-only. A few weeks after they first had intercourse he called: "I have something to tell you...I've been with a girl who has just called me and said that she just found out she has chlamydia, and that I ought to get checked." That there was another girl was a bad enough surprise for Donna; that an STD might be present was even worse.

The moral of this story: know your partner well. Don't assume your relationship is "one-and-only"; talk about it! And then you must depend upon your partner's honesty and resolve. Remember: You can get an STD from a single intimate contact with someone who has it, whether that person realizes he/she is infected or not.

And there's more to be concerned about. All STDs are serious, but teens continue to be infected with HIV disease at an alarming rate. Since the first reports of HIV/AIDS in the early 1980s, HIV/AIDS has become a worldwide epidemic affecting not only homosexual men, but heterosexual men and women, adolescents, children and even infants. Among causes of death in the 25- to 44-year age group, HIV/AIDS is first.

When do you think those 25-year-olds got AIDS? The long incubation period between infection with HIV and diagnosis of AIDS means that most young adults who have it got infected during their teens. Of all new HIV infections in the United States, 25 percent are estimated to occur in young people under the age of 22. AIDS is the sixth leading cause of death for 15- to 24-year-olds in the United States.

The precautions we've listed above for avoiding STDs also apply to staying free from infection with HIV. Don't take chances. You may think that HIV is something that "other people" get; "other people" could be you if you don't take precautions to protect yourself.

Getting tested for an STD requires a trip to a clinic or doctor's office for a physical examination. If an STD is suspected, the clinician will do one or more of the following types of tests. Blood tests are used for STDs such as HIV and syphilis. Microscopic examination of material from genital discharges or lesions, obtained with a cotton swab, are used to identify bacteria under the microscope, such as in the case of chlamydia. Gonorrhea is diagnosed using a culture, for which a swab of secretion from the genital area is placed in a special plate that allows any living bacteria or protozoa to grow and be examined for presence of disease.

Some people are afraid of anybody finding out they have an STD, especially HIV/AIDS. Many STD clinics provide confidential and/or anonymous HIV/AIDS testing — you don't have to provide your name; they just assign you a case number. If you test positive, it's important that you notify your sexual partners so they can be tested, too. If you need assistance locating a place for HIV testing, there are many hotlines and other helpful resources. (See the resources section of this book.)

Below is an overview of STDs that includes descriptions, symptoms, treatment, and consequences of not getting treatment. The basic message is, get tested promptly if there is any chance you've been exposed to an STD; get treated if you have one. For the curable conditions, sexual abstinence is important until the treatment is over and the symptoms clear up. Your doctor or a local health or family planning clinic can provide testing and treatment.

HIV/AIDS

Description and occurrence: Human immunodeficiency virus, or HIV, leads to Acquired Immunodeficiency Syndrome (AIDS). This usually fatal and still incurable illness first appeared in the 1980s. Much has been learned in the past few years about its nature and patterns of transmission. Early in the epidemic many people were worried that they could get HIV simply by being in the same room as someone with the disease, which of course is not true. HIV is spread in blood, semen and vaginal fluids by vaginal and anal intercourse, and oral sex. It is also transmitted by contaminated needles and blood transfusions with contaminated blood. HIV can also be transmitted from a mother to her baby during pregnancy — in about one fourth to one third of cases — and through breastfeeding. HIV is *not* spread by casual contact such as handshakes, hugs, using someone's fork or glass, or toilet seats.

Once in the body, HIV attacks and destroys white blood cells called T-lymphocytes that normally protect us against bacterial, viruses and other microorganisms that we are exposed to daily. The immune system weakens over time as the HIV increases and the number of lymphocytes decreases. A person is considered to have developed AIDS when he or she has less than a certain number of T-cells left. The average time interval between HIV infection and the onset of AIDS is approximately 10 years. The median life expectancy after being infected with HIV is about 12 years, but newly developed drugs are likely to increase that number.

Evidently, people who already have an STD are at greater risk for contracting HIV. It is probably easier for HIV to enter the body through irritated genital tissue and sores.

The body usually reacts to infection by producing antibody proteins against it. The test for HIV/AIDS can detect HIV antibodies in your blood. Current blood tests are over 99 percent accurate. However, it can take from a few days to several months for enough antibodies to develop to be detected in a blood test. For that reason, if your test is negative but you still suspect (or know) that you were exposed to HIV, you need to get tested again a few months later. Meanwhile, take precautions — avoid sexual intercourse or, if you do have sex, use latex condoms — to reduce the risk to others and yourself.

Make sure that the place you go to get tested provides pre- and post-test counseling. A trained counselor can explain to you how the test works and what a negative or positive result means before the test. He or she will go over your results with your after the test. If you test positive, they can refer you for treatment right away; if you are negative, they can discuss with you ways to avoid becoming infected in the future.

Recently, home test kits for HIV have become available. Manufacturers believed that more people might get tested if they could do so anonymously and in the privacy of their own home. These tests, with names such as Confide and Home Access, are available without a prescription at pharmacies, and some can be mailed to you if you call the manufacturers' toll-free numbers. They are the same tests as those in clinics, hospitals and doctors' offices. The kits contain all the supplies you'll need to prick your finger and prepare a blood sample for analysis. You send the sample to a laboratory in a secure mailer, which contains only an ID number so you can remain anonymous. Seven days later, you call in with your ID number and get your test results. There is some controversy surrounding home tests for HIV because of the way the results are provided — over the phone, instead of face-to-face as in doctors' offices or clinics. Someone who gets a negative test result could hang up the phone before they get important information about prevention or the warning that the virus may not have showed up because the test was too soon after exposure, while someone who tests positive may be too distraught to be effectively counseled on the telephone.

We recommend an in-person test with counseling, but recognize that there are some people who might not be tested at all unless they can do it in their own homes.

Symptoms: There are usually none, at first. An HIV-infected person may have flu-like symptoms, such as fever, in the first few days after infection. It is usually after several years as the immune system weakens, that the infected person gets illnesses that healthy people would usually fight off. Among general symptoms are chronic fatigue, weight loss, skin rashes, diarrhea, lung infections, and mental changes.

Treatment: No cure exists for HIV or AIDS, but medications have been developed that help infected people live longer. These include Zidovudine (AZT) and a group of drugs called "protease inhibitors" that can lower the level of virus in the blood. Researchers are also working to develop an AIDS vaccine. It would work by producing antibodies before HIV attacks, giving the body resistance just as measles and polio vaccines do for those illnesses.

CHLAMYDIA

Description and occurrence: Chlamydia is the most common bacterial STD in the United States, infecting 4 million people annually. It is very common among teenagers and young adults. Because chlamydia is often asymptomatic (produces no symptoms) many infected people spread the disease before they even know they have it.

Symptoms: Men may have painful burning sensation while urinating, or watery or milky discharge from the penis. They may also have discomfort in the lower abdomen or testicles during intercourse. Women may have abnormal vaginal discharge, irregular vaginal bleeding, pelvic pain accompanied by nausea and fever, and painful or frequent urination. As mentioned, symptoms may not appear for a long time, and many people never have them. The infection can be spread to the eyes as well, including to the eyes of newborns delivered by women with cervical chlamydia.

Treatment: Chlamydia is curable with antibiotics. Tetracycline and doxycycline are often prescribed.

Consequences if left untreated: In women chlamydia can cause pelvic inflammatory disease (PID), which can lead to sterility, ectopic pregnancy and chronic pelvic pain. In men it can travel up the urethra and infect the spermatic cords and testicles. It can also lead to Reiter's syndrome, in which arthritis and conjunctivitis are major complications.

GONORRHEA

Description and occurrence: In 1994, approximately 800,000 cases of gonorrhea were reported in the United States. Although rates of this bacterial infection have gone down among adolescents over the past few years, in 1993 teenagers ages 15–19 had the highest rate among women and the second highest among men. Nearly half of the patients with gonorrhea are also infected with chlamydia.

Symptoms: There may be none; when they do appear it is usually a few days to a few weeks after exposure. Women may have abnormal vaginal discharge, pelvic pain, unusual vaginal bleeding, bleeding after sex, or swelling or tenderness of the vulva. Men may have burning sensation during urination, milky discharge, or painful sex. Gonorrhea can infect the rectum, throat, and eyes.

Tests for the presence of gonococcus include microscopic examination of cells taken from the urethral area (men) or the cervical area (women), including a cell culture grown on a special plate for up to two days. New, more rapid tests are available but they may be less accurate than the culture.

Treatment: Gonorrhea is curable with antibiotics. Penicillin used to be the best treatment for gonorrhea, but the germ has developed resistance to it and so newer antibiotics, ceftriaxone and doxycycline, are now used.

Consequences if left untreated: In women it can cause pelvic inflammatory disease (PID), which can lead to infertility, ectopic pregnancy and chronic pelvic pain. Men can suffer from infection of the urethra, and disseminated infection can lead to arthritis in men and women. Eye infection in newborns and adults can lead to visual impairment or blindness.

GENITAL WARTS: HUMAN PAPILLOMAVIRUS (HPV)

Description and occurrence: There are over 60 strains of HPV, and estimates are that as many as 50 percent of people in the United States carry at least one. Nearly one million new HPV infections occur each year — many more cases than herpes. In some studies, up to 15 percent of sexually active teen women have been found to be infected with HPV.

The responsible organism is a virus similar to those that cause ordinary warts on the skin. Genital warts occur as small, painless, hard spots on and around the vulva and penis, and around the anus.

Symptoms: Warts may not show up for months or even a year after infection. Women with lesions in the cervix are prone to develop cancer. In addition to the genital area, warts sometimes occur on the anus or throat.

Treatment: There is no cure for the virus. Visible warts can be removed by freezing them with cryosurgery, by applying certain medications, and by electric cautery or surgery.

Consequences if left untreated: HPV is very contagious and will spread. Some strains of HPV are associated with cervical cancer. For that reason, it is important for sexually active young women to get annual Pap smears to test for cervical cancer.

HERPES SIMPLEX

Description and occurrence: Genital herpes is caused by herpes simplex virus types 1 and 2. HSV-1 is usually associated with cold sores around the mouth and HSV-2 with blisters around the genitals, but forms of herpes may be transmitted to the genital area. Approximately 200,000–500,000 new cases occur each year in the United States, and 31 million individuals already are infected. It is estimated that one of every four women and one of every five men in the United States will become infected with herpes during their lifetime.

Symptoms: Itching and soreness usually occur first, then a red sore area or blister develops, which is quite painful. The blister erodes to form a small ulcer. Healing occurs after about ten days. Infections recur because the virus stays dormant and returns to the surface periodically. Many people have no symptoms, but transmission of herpes can occur even when no lesions are present!

Treatment: No cure for herpes has been found, but treatment with medication can help reduce the duration and degree of symptoms. Vaccines are also being developed. Condom use during outbreaks is essential; although transmission is less likely when there are no signs or symptoms, condom use is still advisable to be extra safe.

Consequences if left untreated: Because there is no cure for herpes, both men and women may experience recurrent lesions for years. Treatment may lessen the frequency and severity of the outbreaks.

SYPHILIS

Description and occurrence: There are nearly 100,000 new cases of syphilis each year in this country. This bacterial infection causes a disease that progresses over time by stages (primary, secondary and tertiary), with long intervals (months or years) without any symptoms between them. It can cause permanent damage to many parts of the body, including the brain and heart, if not diagnosed and treated early. Syphilis can be transmitted from a pregnant women to her fetus, causing congenital syphilis, stillbirth, or a baby's death shortly after birth.

Symptoms: Symptoms vary with the stage of the disease. The earliest symptoms include a painless sore (chancre) and enlarged lymph nodes near the chancre. This usually lasts six to ten weeks, and is followed by a latent period that can last from six weeks to six months. By the time the secondary phase is evident, the bacteria have spread throughout the body. Secondary stage symptoms include skin rashes, often followed by another period without symptoms lasting for years.

Finally, tertiary syphilis attacks the nervous system, causing paralysis and mental illness.

Treatment: Antibiotics will cure syphilis if given in the primary, secondary or latent periods. The damage done by tertiary syphilis cannot be reversed.

Consequences if left untreated: Fortunately rare today, tertiary syphilis used to be one of the most common causes of incurable insanity due to lesions in the brain. It also destroys major blood vessels, and causes severe pain in various areas (visceral crises). Congenital syphilis is transmitted through the placenta from mother to baby.

HEPATITIS B

Description and occurrence: This virus affects approximately 200,000 people in the United States each year. About half of the infections are transmitted through sexual intercourse. This is a disease of the liver (from the Greek word *hepatos*) which can cause anything from brief flu-like illness to death.

Symptoms: Early symptoms include nausea, vomiting, fatigue, headache, fever and yellow skin (jaundice).

Treatment: Although there is no cure, in most cases the body repairs itself within several months. A vaccine is available that prevents infection.

Consequences if left untreated: Most cases of Hepatitis B recover after 3 to 4 months, but it can lead to chronic liver disease, cirrhosis, liver cancer and even death.

TRICHOMONIASIS

Description and occurrence: This parasite, the protozoan *Trichomonas*, infects 3 million people each year.

Symptoms: Woman may have vaginal discharge or odor, painful intercourse or frequent urination. Men often do not have symptoms but may experience frequent urination or discharge from the penis.

Treatment: Trichomoniasis is treated with a microbicidal agent called metronidazole, which targets protozoan infections.

Consequences if left untreated: Women will have uncomfortable vaginal discharge. In some cases the vulva and perineum will be inflamed.

CRABS AND SCABIES

Description and occurrence: Pubic lice ("crabs") and scabies (itch mites) are parasites that spread from one person to another through various types of contact, including sexual. Lice attach their eggs to hairs.

Symptoms: Crabs and scabies cause severe itching, which may lead to inflammation.

Treatment: Over-the-counter medications are available as rinses or shampoos. Clothing and bedding must also be decontaminated.

Consequences if left untreated: There is no permanent damage, but itching will persist. If the eyelids and eyelashes become involved, the parasites may have to be removed with forceps.

OTHER STDS

Other diseases transmitted sexually include chancroid, lymphogranuloma venereum, granuloma inguinale, and enteric infections. As we stated earlier, candidiasis (yeast infection) and bacterial vaginosis, common infections among teens, are transmitted sexually in rare instances, but they are not considered sexually transmitted infections. There are more than 25 STDs, at least eight of which are relatively new. We can't cover them all, but you have enough information now to protect yourself and your partner from diseases that range from the merely embarrassing and annoying to the most devastating killers.

> If *every individual* used condoms, along with the spermicidal agent nonoxynol-9 *each* time he or she had sexual intercourse until such time as both partners agreed to enter a permanent, monogamous relationship, AIDS and most other sexually transmitted diseases would begin to vanish from the earth.

So says Stephen L. Sacks, M.D., in *The Truth About Herpes* (3rd ed., 1992, p. 193).

Frequent Asked Questions

Is there any way to determine ahead of time whether a potential sex partner has an STD?

The only way to get an answer to that question is to ask it. Hopefully, you and your partner have built a close enough emotional relationship before having sex to permit an honest exchange of such information. Of course, such checking should be done well in advance of the moment of intercourse. It is a bit unromantic to murmur, "By any chance do you have an STD?" just as you're about to make love. For your physical (and emotional) protection, you may want to ask some general questions about your partner's sexual history and health. You don't have to fire questions like a police officer, but make it your business to know as much about your partner as you can. Of course, you must share the same information about yourself with your partner. You could ask, "Are you sleeping with anyone else?" "Have you had other sexual partners? If so, have you used condoms?" You can even ask if he or she has had an HIV test. But remember that tests may not detect the virus if less than six months have passed since infection. To make the issue less confrontational, you can suggest that you and your partner get tested together.

I know that women can get gonorrhea without showing any symptoms. Can the same thing happen to men?

Yes. Asymptomatic gonorrhea (gonorrhea with no symptoms) can occur in both men and women. Any suspicion of exposure should be followed by a test at a doctor's office or clinic.

If you get an STD, you're supposed to tell everyone you've had sex with. How do you tell someone something like that?

It's not easy, but it's important. In fact, all states require contact tracing and reporting of cases for syphilis and gonorrhea. Some states have additional reporting requirements for other STDs. Contact tracing means notifying the sexual partners of an infected person so they can also get examined and treated for the disease. States also require that health professionals report the number of cases of gonorrhea and chlamydia to public health officials so they can track trends and allocate resources as necessary. Don't let these reporting requirements keep you from getting tested and treated if you have an STD. Health clinic counselors can help you plan the best way to tell your partner, or they can even do it for you if you choose.

Telling someone is no easy matter, but the damage from the spread of AIDS, or even a case of untreated gonorrhea, means that prevention and early treatment can literally save lives. Put yourself in your partner's position — wouldn't you want to be told? Besides, if you don't tell your partner, then even if you get treated you may catch the disease again since your partner may still have it!

Before telling, do a bit of psychological preparation. Think about the fact that you're doing something honest, considerate and necessary. Also be aware that the earlier you catch and treat STDs, the less the damage. Then consider what makes you most uncomfortable and what will make it easier for your partner to deal with the news. Does a phone conversation seem easier than meeting in person? What if he or she takes your call when others are present? Under no circumstances should you leave a message on an answering machine (where someone else could hear it) or with a roommate. That's not only cowardly, it's cruel. Even if you are angry at the other person because you're sure that's where you got infected, remember: It takes two to spread those germs.

I had sex with Kurt, who I know has been with lots of girls. I think I should probably get an HIV test, but I'm afraid to find out I have HIV. What should I do?

You're right to think you should get an HIV test — having sex with someone who has had multiple partners (or even one other partner) is a risk factor for contracting HIV. As scary as it is to get tested and possibly learn that you do have HIV, it is the right thing to do for several reasons. First, you will very likely find out you don't have HIV; that would give you a "second chance" to be more careful. Second, if you test positive, you will be able to protect your health and that of others better by knowing. Remember that the HIV test may not detect HIV soon after exposure. If you test negative and less than six months have passed since exposure, get tested again later.

Chapter 4

Condoms—His and Hers

Why does it take 300,000,000 sperm to fertilize one egg? Because none of them will stop and ask for directions.

Actually, it takes only one sperm to fertilize an egg. But each ejaculation releases hundreds of millions of sperm in about a teaspoon of semen (sperm plus seminal fluid).

The male condom — also called "sheath" or "rubber"— is designed to contain all the sperm, preventing any from reaching an egg. Since the condom envelops the penis from tip to base, it also keeps germs (bacteria, viruses) in or out: The male may have them in the urethra or on the penis, while the female may carry them inside the vagina, or outside on the vulva. In the age of HIV/AIDS, preventing the spread of disease is a matter of life and death whether in a heterosexual or homosexual relationship.

"Condom" used to be a dirty word. Now it is known as a lifesaver, a vital factor in public health and preventive medicine. Condom vending machines can be found more frequently. The condom has many names: "rubber," "prophylactic" (something that protects or guards), and "preservativo" (Spanish); the French call it "la capote anglaise" ("English cape") and in England it has been called "the French letter."

A thin sheath of latex rubber, animal membrane (nicknamed "skins") or polyurethane plastic, the condom is the one contraceptive that prevents infection as well as pregnancy. A female condom has recently been marketed; we will discuss it later.

One of the best first methods of contraception for most people, the male condom is the one most frequently used by teens for many reasons. Preparing for sex makes for a better relationship: Taking precautions is more loving than being "swept away." Experienced lovers know that good sex combines forethought and spontaneity — it is not impulsive or mindless but rather imaginative and caring.

When a couple has experienced sexual arousal and feel that intercourse is a possibility, *they should talk about it.* Sexual consideration — with contraception — is more deeply caring and more truly romantic than unplanned surprises. You don't learn this from TV or movies, but sex gets better when it is planned, anticipated, prepared for — like many of the best things in life. Inexperienced lovers are aware of the excitement that goes with sex, but they must learn that a relaxed atmosphere is essential for a good sexual relationship. Hurrying and anxiety, guilt and embarrassment — all interfere. Worry about pregnancy and STDs can ruin the sexual experience, especially for women.

A recent study in the Detroit area found that young women 16 and older did almost as well with condom use as adult women: 80 percent used one at last intercourse. That's good, but not good enough.

> Marla, a 16-year-old student, has never had intercourse. "I feel it is up to my boyfriend Brad to use a condom," she said. "Why should I have to make an appointment to get the pill or something when he can get condoms at the drug store? As a woman I'll probably be taking birth control responsibility for most of my life. I think the guy should assume the responsibility, at least at first." Brad agrees: "If we decide to have sex, it's up to me to help make sure she doesn't get pregnant."
>
> * * *
>
> Linda, a student who is also 16, explained that she and her boyfriend decided to rely on the condom because they do not have sex that often. "The condom makes the most sense for us. Why should I take a pill every day when we only have sex once or twice a month?"

Although we do not think that teens — or anyone — should have multiple partners or casual sex, it does happen. Condoms are a must under those circumstances.

> Paul is 18, a high school senior, and plays the stud. He doesn't want to "belong" to just one girl. He makes a point of playing the field, dating — or just bedding — a different girl every few

weeks. "I don't know which girls are using what precautions," he says, "or who they've slept with. You never know what diseases are out there. Better safe than sorry. You need protection and the condom is it."

Sexual "hype" in the media is designed to attract an audience, not teach about responsible behavior. It's not easy to make caution and prevention exciting: They get in the way of the story. On TV and in the movies, sex is all about feeling, not much about thinking. Condoms don't fit the myth that lovers are just swept away with passion.

There is nothing wrong with great romance, but Hollywood stories usually omit the part about common sense. How many conversations about birth control have you heard on soap operas? And how many discussions about AIDS have you heard during prime time TV bedroom scenes? How can we believe a couple is prepared with contraception if they've never discussed it?

History and Background

According to one story, the condom was named for its inventor, a Doctor Condom, court physician to Charles II of England in the seventeenth century. The story, long held but now in doubt, has it that the device became so famous that the doctor changed his name.

Early versions of the condom date back many centuries: Animal bladders were used in ancient Rome, and condoms were thought of as a barrier against syphilis long before its transmission by microbes was understood.

Some of the earliest condoms were made from dried sheep gut. Those are still known as "skins." While these became popular as a way to prevent pregnancy, they did not protect well against disease because viruses and bacteria are small enough to pass through the membrane (sperm are much larger).

The modern condom became possible with the invention in 1844 of a rubber-making process called vulcanization (named for the ancient Roman god of fire and metalworking). Only then could the bouncy, gummy stuff (named for its use in rubbing out pencil mistakes) be made stretchy and strong. Vulcanization revolutionized the rubber industry;

condoms became better, cheaper, and much more popular. Condoms were further improved in the 1930s when they could be made of latex, a thinner and stronger rubber product. In 1938, the U.S. Food and Drug Administration began setting and enforcing standards for condom quality.

In the 1950s and 1960s condom use declined for two reasons. First, penicillin and other antibiotics were found to be effective in treating syphilis and gonorrhea. Second, the contraceptive pill became the most popular method of birth control — both men and women preferred it to the condom. In the 1980s HIV/AIDS brought back the condom. Next to abstinence, the latex condom is the best means of preventing the spread of HIV/AIDS. Between 1982 and 1990, condom use increased sharply among teenagers, from 21 to 44 percent.

How It Works

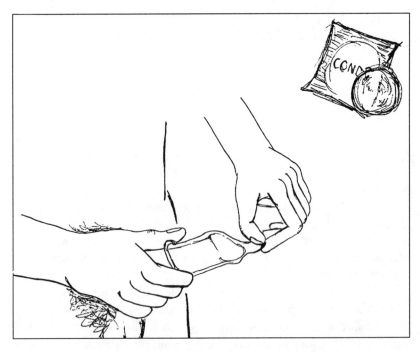

Figure 1: Male condom: Roll on (and off) holding ring. Make space at tip.

A man puts on a condom by carefully unrolling it onto the erect penis. It is similar to the way women put on good stockings or panty-hose, with one difference: Leave the condom a little slack at the tip, not snug like the toe of a stocking. Some condoms have a reservoir tip to catch the semen (you don't have to worry about leaving slack at the end). With the regular kind you must gently pinch the tip to get any air out and leave room for the ejaculate (about a teaspoonful of semen).

The open end of the condom has a rubber ring that keeps it in place at the base of the penis. Either partner can hold the ring when withdrawing after vaginal, anal or even oral sex.

There are plain or lubricated (slippery) latex condoms and "skins" made from lamb membranes. Polyurethane condoms (plastic) came on the market more recently. Some condoms are coated with a spermicide called nonoxynol-9 that promises some extra protection against pregnancy, though no one is certain just how much. Condoms also come in different colors, textures, and flavors (for oral sex). Beware of the colors: Some people are allergic to the dyes that are used. And remember: A condom should be used only once and then discarded.

Condoms, carefully and consistently used, are very effective in preventing pregnancy. However, *only condoms made out of latex protect against STDs*. Natural membrane condoms, "skins," have microscopic pores large enough to let through syphilis and gonorrhea bacteria, and the much smaller herpes and AIDS viruses. (Viruses are the smallest living things.) Testing of the polyurethane condom's effectiveness is still underway.

Getting and Using It

Condoms are sold in most drug stores, with no prescription needed. Condoms may still be kept behind pharmacy counters, but usually they are available with other personal products. Condoms are also often sold at grocery stores, and in some restrooms from vending machines. Planned Parenthood, neighborhood health clinics, and some school-based health centers also distribute condoms, sometimes for a charge and sometimes for free.

Learning how to use a condom correctly only takes a minute (men can even practice by themselves). After the male is aroused (penis erect) but *before any genital contact*, put on the condom. Why so soon? Because

(1) HIV cells are present in the pre-ejaculate (the small amount of fluid that is released from the penis before ejaculation) of HIV-infected men;

(2) ejaculation may occur sooner than expected; and

(3) infection can spread if genital contact occurs without the condom.

Condoms come rolled up in individual packages. Open the package carefully. (Teeth or a scissors can tear the rubber.) The condom rolls easily over the erect penis (uncircumcised males should first pull back the foreskin), but leave a half-inch of space at the tip to collect the semen (make sure the space is not filled with air, or the tip could burst like a bubble). The rubber ring goes all the way to the base.

Ideally, the woman's sexual arousal produces vaginal secretions that provide lubrication and make penetration easy. Sometimes another lubricant will be necessary. Latex condoms should also be used during anal intercourse to protect against HIV. Condoms are more likely to tear during anal intercourse than vaginal intercourse, but using a generous amount of lubricant helps avoid tearing. With latex condoms, use only water-based lubricants, such as contraceptive cream or K-Y jelly (glycerin) or even saliva. *Never* use petroleum jelly and mineral oil products, such as baby oil, cold cream, Vaseline, or many hand lotions: They make rubber deteriorate.

Soon after intercourse, before the penis gets soft, grasp the condom firmly at the base and withdraw the penis. It is important to do this before the erection has gone down so that none of the seminal fluid trapped inside the condom leaks out. If the male loses his erection before climax (it sometimes happens), he must carefully and promptly withdraw because the condom no longer fits tightly. The condom is secure and effective only with a firm erection.

Condoms can last for several years in their original packages, but they can be ruined if they are carried around in a pocket or wallet, or left in a car, where they may be damaged by high temperatures if the car is left parked in the sun. Before using a condom, check to see that its foil wrapping or other packaging is unbroken. If the package is damaged, or you suspect that the condom may have been damaged, do not use it. Different brands date their condoms differently, but you can use the information on the package to get an idea of the condom's age. Condoms that contain spermicide have a shelf life of roughly two or three years (to assure the spermicide still works), while other condoms last as many as five years on the shelf. The general rule is that if you have any doubt about the condition of a condom, throw it out and get a new one. Better safe than sorry.

Being prepared with a condom is a problem for some. Couples should talk about sex before they have it, but many do not. For many people sex is easier to do than to talk about. Neither partner may want to appear prepared or over-eager, though each has unspoken thoughts or hopes about having sex. If a boy has a condom ready, the girl may feel insulted: "He takes me for granted!" If the girl brings a condom the boy thinks, "She is doing my job, and it makes me feel insecure!" Just because the male wears the condom doesn't mean the female can't share in the responsibility for safer sex and provide the condom once in a while.

What about the inconvenience of using a condom? Creative couples have found ways to turn application of the condom into foreplay (some couples may take a while before becoming this comfortable with each other). Males who are concerned that the condoms will reduce sensation can try some of the brands that claim to enhance sensitivity. Condoms can also help in another way: Less sensation allows longer lovemaking for the man.

Effectiveness

The latex condom is an excellent contraceptive and prophylactic (preventive) against STDs. How often do they fail?

Used with perfect technique, condoms fail only two percent of the time. In ordinary use, the failure rate is about 12 percent: 12 out of 100 women will become pregnant in a year. This is still quite respectable, since with no method 85 percent would become pregnant.

These statistics show how important it is to use the condom properly. Most condom failures are due to improper, careless or inconsistent use, not to a defect in the material. Breakage rates are less than two percent, and most breakage is due to incorrect use rather than poor quality of the condom. Failure can occur without breakage if semen leaks out of the open end. (Women can become pregnant due to sperm being deposited quite low down in the vagina — this explains some "virgin" pregnancies, when a male ejaculates during sex play, even though intercourse never took place.) Petroleum products also break down latex quickly enough to allow semen to seep through.

One way to increase the effectiveness of the condom against pregnancy is to use it with a spermicide. Some condoms are coated with a spermicide, usually nonoxynol-9; it is not known whether this makes a difference if the condom breaks. Adding more spermicide can also help. And, of course, combining the condom with other contraceptive methods, such as the diaphragm, boosts effectiveness.

Safety and Side Effects

Condoms are in a class by themselves when it comes to safety. Unless a man or his partner has an allergy to latex, there are no side effects. If allergy to latex is a problem, try the female condom or the plastic male condom.

Some males say condoms block sensation. We hear objections such as, "Guys don't like them. They say 'It doesn't feel natural,' or 'I don't want to be cooped up,' or 'It's like taking a shower with a raincoat on.'"

If he cares about his relationship — his partner and himself — a man will take precautions. Beware of guys making excuses not to use a condom. They may be too embarrassed to buy them, or just selfish (men don't get pregnant). Some men may even try to prove their "manhood" by making girls pregnant. If this is what makes a guy feel masculine, watch out.

Sometimes a woman will object to a condom, saying it hurts or doesn't feel right. Inadequate lubrication can be a problem, and a lubricant might help.

The Condom and STDs

It bears repeating that latex condoms offer significant protection against sexually transmitted diseases (STDs). Natural membrane condoms do not, since they are more porous and allow microorganisms — bacteria, viruses, tiny parasites — to pass through. It will be a few years before we know how effective plastic condoms are in protecting against STDs and pregnancy.

All sexually transmitted diseases are serious and some are deadly, such as HIV/AIDS. Many efforts to prevent the spread of HIV/AIDS have focused on convincing sexually active people to use condoms. This applies not only to sexual intercourse, but to oral and anal sex. Bodily fluids, which spread the virus, are exchanged in those situations. The same rules for condom use apply for oral sex and anal sex: Put it on before any contact occurs.

The bottom line is that next to abstinence, or staying mutually faithful with a partner who is not a carrier of disease, using a condom is the best protection available against the spread of STDs.

The Female Condom

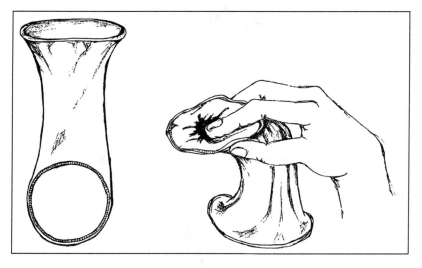

Figure 2: Female condom.

The latest condom development is the "female condom," called "Reality" in the United States. Like the male condom, it does not require fitting by a health care professional and is available in drug stores and other retail outlets wherever condoms for men are sold. They cost about $2.25 each. The female condom is a loose-fitting polyurethane sheath with one closed end that the woman inserts deep inside the vagina. The open end remains outside the vagina and is entered by the penis. The sheath provides a physical barrier between partners during sexual intercourse protecting them from each other's bodily fluids. It is sold with its own lubricant and has a shelf life of three years. Each should be used once and discarded.

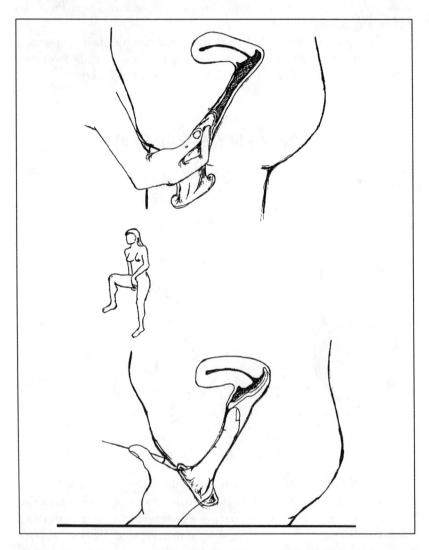

Figure 3 (top): Female condom insertion. Figure 4 (bottom): Insertion completed.

To use the female condom, squeeze the inner ring between your fingers and insert it into the vagina. Push the inner ring up until it is just behind the pubic bone. About an inch of the open end should be outside your body. Right after ejaculation, squeeze and twist the outer ring and pull the pouch out gently. Like the male condom, it should be used only once and then discarded. As with other barrier methods, it's a good idea to practice inserting "Reality" by yourself before using it with your partner.

One advantage of the "Reality" condom is that it can be inserted ahead of time so that sexual intercourse is not interrupted. Once in place, the prelubricated condom adheres to the vaginal wall, so the penis can move freely. Some couples need extra lubrication. Putting a few drops on the penis or at the condom's opening helps reduce friction. Because "Reality" is made of plastic instead of latex (like most condoms for men), you can use both oil- and water-based lubricants with it. It should *not* be used with a male condom.

"Reality" was developed by a Danish physician who was concerned about transmission of STDs and felt that women needed a protective method to use themselves. Initial studies found a pregnancy rate of 26 percent, significantly higher than for other barrier methods. However, more recent research has found pregnancy rates declining to 18–25 percent for typical use and 5 percent for "perfect use." Improvements may be due to the fact that women are getting more used to them.

We don't know yet how effective the female condom is in protecting against STDs. But it appears that female condoms, used properly, provide more protection than male condoms because they cover a greater area, offering better protection against herpes and warts, for example. Additional studies are underway.

Conclusion

The latex condom is probably the best first method of birth control for most people, not just teens. Condoms are safe and effective for preventing pregnancy and sexually transmitted diseases. They are easier to get and to use compared to the most effective female methods (pill and Norplant). Couples can choose other methods of birth control as their sexual relationship becomes established. Even so, using a condom along with another method of birth control offers extra protection against pregnancy and STDs.

The condom is the one method that allows men to take responsibility for birth control and hygiene. Most of the time women take responsibility for preventing pregnancy. If a woman is pressured to go on the pill because her partner is too shy or stubborn to use a condom, she'll probably be resentful, not a good way to start or keep an intimate relationship. Latex condoms are a good first method for most young couples and are always good for combining with other methods for added protection.

Frequently Asked Questions

Can I just walk into any drug store and buy condoms?

Yes. There are no laws or restrictions regarding the selling of condoms to teenagers. You can buy them wherever they are sold, including supermarkets and vending machines. They are usually displayed in an accessible area near other personal products. If you go to a store where a cashier or pharmacist is not helpful, another store will be glad to have you as a customer. Also, Planned Parenthood and other clinics provide condoms at very low prices, or even free. Condoms may also be ordered through the mail and via the Internet.

Can girls buy condoms?

Yes, they can and they do. A girl may want to share the expense or just take the initiative for a change. Women can now buy the female condom ("Reality") in drug stores — and so can men.

Why are condoms less than 100 percent effective in preventing pregnancy?

To be effective, a condom has to be in good condition and used properly. If the package is open a long time, or takes a beating in someone's pocket, or is in contact with a petroleum product such as Vaseline, it will be weakened. A condom can break if the user fails to leave about half an inch of slack space at the tip to catch the semen. A condom can slip off if the penis is not withdrawn from the vagina or anus while it is still erect. Very rarely is a condom defective when bought. Human error is the main reason that condoms sometimes fail.

Can a condom be reused?

Condoms — male and female — are not meant to be reused. The smart couple always has two; if one condom seems defective (rare), there's a spare. More importantly, young couples often want to have intercourse more than once on the same occasion.

What if the condom doesn't fit?

Men of all shapes and sizes have used condoms of all styles for decades without problem. Condoms come in different shapes and slightly different sizes, but one size fits all: "Large" is designed only to fit big male egos. Any man who says a condom doesn't fit either does not know how to put one on properly, or doesn't want to.

Why do some couples use foam or jelly with condoms?

That helps take care of the small percentage of occasions when condoms fail; combining contraceptives increases your protection. Also, since condoms are the primary method for preventing the transmission of STDs, using them with other birth control methods that don't protect against STDs, such as the pill, makes sense.

What happens if the condom breaks or falls off?

If that happens, the girl should call Planned Parenthood, a similar clinic, or her doctor within 24 hours. They can decide whether emergency contraception would be appropriate. Both homosexual and heterosexual couples should talk about getting tested for HIV/AIDS or other STDs if there is a chance that one partner exposed the other.

I've used condoms before, but my girlfriend says she doesn't want to use a condom for our "first time."

Some people think you can't get pregnant the first time. They're wrong. You can tell her the condom won't interfere with the closeness of your experience together, that it's a minor — but important — part of a major experience. If she balks, ask her to visit her doctor or a clinic to get another reliable contraceptive. Beware of a girl who doesn't seem worried about pregnancy or STDs. She or you may suddenly wake up in a panic when it's too late.

What about using plastic food wrap if you don't have a condom?

Lots of creative methods have been tried — and failed. Sex is never an emergency, so why risk ruining two (or more) lives by taking a chance?

Don't condoms block sensations?

Physically, a little. Psychologically, the only feeling condoms interfere with is the one you can do without: anxiety about pregnancy and infection. To the extent that the condom filters the male's skin sensations during foreplay and thrusting, it gives him more control. He will still reach the peak of excitement and pleasure (orgasm), so he has nothing to complain about. His ability to take more time enables him to give his partner more pleasure. In an established relationship, when he has good control during sex, when she is ready to assume responsibility for birth control, and when the risk of STDs is zero, then it may be nice to choose another method.

I went to see my doctor after experiencing vaginal burning and pain after intercourse. She told me I was probably allergic to latex. I understand that nonlatex condoms don't protect against STDs. Is there any good alternative to latex condoms?

Latex allergies are becoming more common. There is no perfect solution to your problem, but there are some steps you can take. You can use the female condom, which is made of polyurethane. Although we don't know how effective it is in protecting against STDs, it is better than using no protection. Or you can use two male condoms. Since you have the allergy to latex, your partner should first put on a latex condom (to protect against STDs) and then put on the natural membrane condom (to protect you from the latex). If it's the man who has the latex allergy, reverse the arrangement and put the "skin" condom on first. Using two condoms at once is not usually recommended because the friction of one rubbing against the other might cause tears, or pull them off. But latex allergy is one situation where using two male condoms makes sense. Do not use a male and female condom together because the friction will damage both.

Can spermicide be used with Reality, the female condom?

Yes. Although studies on this have not been completed, common sense suggests that it's a good idea. The spermicide should be inserted into the vagina before putting in the condom.

Chapter 5

The Pill

Human beings are mammals, which means we are warm-blooded, have hair, and nurse our young (*mamma* is Latin for "breast"). Sex among mammals is controlled by a complicated system of hormones. For most mammals — but not humans — the female is receptive to the male only when an egg is ready to be fertilized. This is because the goal of sex for them is pregnancy and procreation. This brief window of opportunity for sex is signaled to the male of most mammal species by a chemical (pheromone) emitted by the female: Without the signal he's not interested; when it's there, he can think of little else.

Humans are different. The female's egg is ready only once a month for a day or so, but sex can happen any time. Males are interested regardless of pheromones. Human sex happens for reasons besides desire for pregnancy, namely love, intimacy and pleasure.

The birth control pill closes the window of opportunity to get pregnant. Those few days of fertility don't happen. The woman does not ovulate (produce an egg) because the hormone contained in the pill signals the pituitary gland to hold off, as though the woman were already pregnant.

The oral contraceptive, often referred to as "the pill," was a major development in birth control in the 1960s. The pill was a more convenient and effective method of birth control than had ever before been available to women.

In the three decades since its discovery, the pill has had problems, been redesigned, yet remains very popular. Some like it more than others. Properly used, it provides nearly perfect contraception, but it is not for everyone.

Alice, 18, started taking the pill shortly after she and her boy-friend, Sam, started having sexual intercourse. "We were using condoms at first," said Sam. "But after a while we got tired of having to stop everything and put it on." "I decided to try the pill instead," said Alice. "I really like it — I just take it when I wake up each morning and we know we're set. It's so conve-nient."

* * *

Jackie and her boyfriend David, both 17, talked about contra-ception before having sex. Jackie decided to try going on the pill. "I hated it," she said. "I didn't feel good about taking these pills every day when we were only having sex, like, once a week or something. Why should I have to mess with my whole body chemistry for that?" David liked the pill. "To me it seemed really convenient. But Jackie was really unhappy about it, so she's going to try the diaphragm instead."

An important limitation of the pill is that it does not protect the user from sexually transmitted diseases (STDs) such as HIV/AIDS. So everyone who uses the pill should consider using latex condoms when there is any risk of exposure to STDs.

History and Background

Birth control advocate Margaret Sanger (1883–1966), who fought relentlessly for legalized contraception, and Katherine Dexter McCor-mick, who financed the entire research effort that produced the oral contraceptive, are considered the mothers of the pill. It has had several "fathers," too, including John Rock, M.D., an obstetrician-gynecolo-gist who made important discoveries while searching for the key to fer-tility. His goal was to help women who were infertile (i.e., having trou-ble getting pregnant).

Dr. Rock built on prior discoveries about the reproductive cycle and the hormones that control it. As he figured out how to control the mechanisms that assist conception, he realized that the same mecha-nisms could be used to block conception. Over the years Rock and his colleagues tried giving various levels of progesterone and estrogen to animals — and later to humans — to keep the ovaries from releasing an egg each month. Large-scale field testing began in family planning clinics in Puerto Rico in 1955. It took only six years from the first animal tests to a worldwide prescription boom in which millions of women were taking the pill daily. It was approved by the U.S. Food and Drug Administration (FDA) on May 11, 1960.

John Rock always stressed that this revolutionary development was a team effort. Other scientists associated with the pill include Gregory Pincus, C. M. Garcia and Carl Djerassi. Developing the pill was only half the battle. The other half was having it accepted by the world, which meant overcoming objections from the Catholic church. Dr. Rock, a Roman Catholic himself, hoped the oral contraceptive would not be opposed by the church, but he was to be disappointed. (The Catholic church opposes it still.) Nevertheless, his concerns about the dangers of over-population and the tragedy of unwanted pregnancy turned him into an unrelenting advocate for the pill. As a result, the pill stands as one of the most important medical discoveries of modern times. It is seen as a blessing by women of many faiths from all over the world, including many Catholics.

How It Works

Ordinarily a woman's ovaries release one egg (ovum or ova [plural]); every 28 days or so (ovulation), in response to a hormone signal. The pill stops this signal by producing a chemical imitation of pregnancy. The pituitary (master gland) in the brain withholds the signal to the body to go through the monthly fertility cycle. The woman does not ovulate and therefore cannot become pregnant, even if sperm enter her body, because no egg is available.

There are two kinds of oral contraceptives: the combination pill, which contains both hormones estrogen and progestin; and the mini-pill, which contains only progestin. The combination pill is much more common, so we devote most of this chapter to it. Besides inhibiting ovulation, it works in two other ways to prevent pregnancy. It causes the cervix to produce a thicker mucus that sperm cells cannot easily penetrate; and it keeps the lining of the uterus from filling out as it usually does between ovulation and menstruation. If somehow an egg were to be released and fertilized, the thin lining keeps that egg from implanting itself in the uterus.

The minipill is used by women who cannot tolerate estrogen. They are very low-dose, which makes them slightly less effective than combination pills. Like combination pills, they provide no protection against STDs.

Many brands of combination pills are available. Some combine hormones in a single pill, while others provide them in sequence. Some are taken for 21 days per cycle and others for 28 days. They come in plastic cases, circular dial packs, or cameo compacts with calendar numbers to help you keep on schedule.

Getting and Using It

The pill is a prescription item and must be obtained from a physician or clinic. Each state has parental consent and notification rules for medical care for minors, including rules for prescribing medications. All states but one permit minors to seek contraceptives on their own (Utah restricts state family planning money). However, a physician may insist on parent notification anyway; so, if that matters, ask about your doctor's policy before making an appointment for contraception.

Most women feel comfortable asking their own doctors about the pill; teenagers may be reluctant to ask their life-long pediatrician or family practitioner. But all sexually active girls should have a gynecological exam. Each person has to evaluate her own situation and make the decision as to where she is most comfortable getting care — a family planning clinic or a private doctor's office, for example.

If you prefer a private physician to a clinic doctor and want to be sure that the physician you choose will be helpful, you can do two things: Ask your mother, sister, aunt, or a girlfriend who takes the pill to recommend a doctor; or simply phone a physician's office and ask the receptionist, "Does the doctor prescribe birth control, including the pill, for teenagers?" If the answer is "no," ask for a referral to another doctor. If the answer is "yes," ask for an appointment. You might also ask about cost, since private practitioners often charge more than Planned Parenthood and publicly-supported family planning clinics.

You should not lie about your age, pretend to be married, or go though any charades to get the pill. *Never* use someone else's prescription. A doctor needs accurate information in order to decide if the pill will be safe and effective for you. In a few cases, the pill can cause serious side effects. Some women may feel more comfortable visiting a Planned Parenthood office or other clinic that has been established for the very purpose of helping with birth control information and services. As one teenager explained:

> People really seem to care about you. They choose to do this work because they believe in it. I got the feeling that some of them have daughters my age. Maybe it's just the experience they have every day with people like me.

All clinics that are funded through Title X [Ten], a federal family planning program, provide contraceptives for teenagers. Under current law, clinics that receive Title X funds are not permitted to notify parents of minor patients that they have provided prescription contraceptives to the teenager; so if you go to one of these clinics, they can't tell your parents. Some school-based clinics offer reproductive health services, and nearly one-fourth of them provide oral contraceptives.

A number of medical organizations have advised that teenage girls should have the same access to birth control as older, married women. In 1971, the influential Executive Board of the American College of Obstetricians and Gynecologists issued an advisory statement saying: "[T]he unmarried female of any age should have access to the most effective forms of contraception ... even in the case of the unemancipated minor who refuses to involve her parents." (An "unemancipated minor" is defined differently in different states, but generally it means a young person who is under the legal age of consent and is not married, self-supporting, or in the Armed Services.)

The physician or other health care provider that you see will ask about your medical history and may do a pelvic examination. Many factors can affect your ability to use the pill: cigarette smoking; varicose veins; family history of diabetes; tendency to form blood clots; liver trouble; heart disease; glandular disease; eye problems; vaginal conditions; skin problems; migraine headaches; epilepsy; and psychiatric problems. Although that may seem like a long list of factors to consider, it is important to make sure that the pill is safe and right for you.

The doctor will also take into account your age, since a younger woman's hormonal patterns may not be well established. In that case, the doctor may recommend using another contraceptive method for the time being. But menstrual irregularity is not always a deterrent; in fact, the pill is sometimes used to help make periods more regular.

If everything is medically normal, and your doctor and you agree that the pill is a good method for you, he or she will prescribe it. The doctor will explain that there are several different kinds of pills, some containing more hormones than others. Some are taken for 21 days each month, and others for 28 days. Your health care provider will tell you when to start taking the pill and will recommend that you use a back-up method of contraception for a period of time until the pill has begun working.

With the 21-day combination pill compact, you follow a "three weeks on, one week off" pattern of pill-taking. You will take a pill every day for 21 days; then, you will take none for seven days while you have your period. Then you begin a new cycle with a new compact.

With 28-day compacts, you take a pill every day of the month. However, you are actually taking birth control pills for only the first 21 days; during the last seven days, which includes your period, the pills contain sugar or iron, not hormones. (They are called "placebos.") Some women find this to be a more convenient schedule since they do not have to remember when to stop and when to start the pills each month — they take a pill every day. There is no medical difference between the 21- and 28-day pills. Minipills are taken every day and there are no placebos.

Your health care provider may give you a prescription for one, three, or more compacts and then advise you to come back for a checkup when you need a new pill supply. It is a good idea not to have the entire prescription filled at once, since you will want to make sure that the particular type of pill you get works well for you. Some women end up switching brands:

> Sixteen-year-old Lorna, for example, was given a pill that contained only a "mini" dose of estrogen. She worried about pregnancy when her periods practically disappeared. This is because she tended to have light periods in the first place, and since the pill keeps the lining of the uterus from becoming very thick, her monthly discharges were lighter than ever. When Lorna

phoned her gynecologist to report this, he explained that if she took the pill regularly, her light periods were not a sign of pregnancy. She could either enjoy the relative ease of very light monthly flow, or if she felt more comfortable with a more normal flow, he would give her a new prescription for a different pill with a higher dose of estrogens. She chose to change.

Lorna's experience points to the importance of answering all questions carefully when you are examined by your doctor. When Lorna had been asked if her periods were normal, she said "Yes," not thinking to mention her light flow. Her experience also points out that a brand of the pill that is right for your best friend may not be the right brand for you. You should not trade pill compacts with friends, nor should you ever accept pills from anyone other than your health care provider.

Whichever brand of pill you're on, it must be taken for a full cycle, as directed. A few girls have had the idea that they could protect themselves from pregnancy by "snitching" just one pill from a friend or older sister's compact and taking it on an evening when they thought they would have sexual intercourse. Not only will this fail to protect the girl who "borrows" the one pill; it messes up the pill owner's schedule as well and puts her at risk of getting pregnant.

Effectiveness

Because the pill acts in several ways to prevent pregnancy, it is highly effective. In typical use, the pill has a failure rate of only five percent per year. With perfect use, that rate drops to less than one percent. A large proportion of oral-contraceptors forget to take their pills consistently; many of them are lucky and don't get pregnant, but many do.

Contraceptive failure can occur if a woman does not use a backup method of birth control for the first packet of pills, or forgets to take a pill for two or more days. Antibiotics and some other medications that are metabolized in the liver interfere with the pill. Be sure and tell your health care provider about all medications you are taking before adding another one.

Safety and Side Effects

The pill is safe when properly prescribed under good medical supervision. Over the past 30 years, millions of girls and women have taken billions of pills, with an excellent record of safety and satisfaction. Like any other drug, of course, the pill is not for everyone. The benefits must be weighed against the risks.

The pill has been closely watched ever since it was introduced. In the early days the pill contained stronger doses of hormones, which raised fears about side effects, including an increased risk of breast cancer. Because the dosages have been lowered, these risks have been greatly reduced.

The pill is also believed to reduce the risk of certain cancers, such as ovarian cancer and uterine cancer. Whether the effect of birth control pills on reproductive cancers is positive or negative, it is probably very small.

The American College of Obstetricians and Gynecologists has concluded that the risks associated with pill use by teenagers are negligible. Low-dose oral contraceptives have not been linked with either heart attacks or stroke in recent studies in the United States. The risk of blood clots (thromboembolism) may be higher for pill users than for other women, but the risk to teenagers — except possibly for those who smoke — is believed to be minimal. The risk of death or disability from oral contraceptives is small, and proper medical screening and supervision make it even smaller.

The pill offers benefits besides contraception. Some women have a more regulated menstrual cycle; some have less menstrual cramps and pain; and some have a clearer complexion.

Unfortunately, the pill also has some undesirable side effects in a few women, as is to be expected with any potent medication. These include slight bleeding ("spotting") between periods, weight gain or fluid retention, breast tenderness, and nausea. These side effects often disappear after about three months of taking the pill. Switching brands of pills may reduce undesirable side effects, and if you have any you should discuss that option with your health care provider.

Should a woman take a break from the pill after a few years? Experts basically agree that women do not need to take a break from the pill. Since the pill stops ovulation, some women find it reassuring to let the body resume regular cycles after several years. Remember to begin using another contraceptive method immediately if you stop taking the pill.

The Pill and STDs

Using a condom along with the pill is a good idea if there is any possibility that one partner is infected. The pill does not prevent transmission of STDs such as HIV/AIDS, herpes or gonorrhea. Approximately ¼ of the 1.7 million teenagers who use the pill also use condoms for this reason.

The pill also changes the chemistry of the vagina enough to favor the growth of certain microorganisms. Some women have minor but annoying vaginal infections from yeast or fungus growth. These respond to simple treatment.

More serious is the problem of gonorrhea. It may have a greater chance of getting established in a woman on the pill than in a woman who is not, assuming exposure to the bacillus. Since most women do not have symptoms in the early stage of gonorrhea, they can harbor the disease and be contagious without knowing it.

Conclusion

Since 1967 the safety of the pill has improved and women who take it do so with greater confidence. Pill users tend to be quite enthusiastic about their choice: "Other methods you just tolerate," said Amy, a 17 year old, "but the pill is an absolute pleasure. To me, that little compact represents absolute security." Many women like the pill because of its convenience. Taking something orally is easier for many than using genital methods. There is nothing to interfere with sensations, and no interruptions of sexual play before intercourse.

However, not everyone is enthusiastic about the pill. Some women have a hard time remembering to take it every day. If you're going through a rough period with your lover or are separated or sexually inactive for a while, taking the pill can be an emotionally charged event and may be forgotten, or omitted on purpose. Noncompliance (not taking medication as prescribed) may be due to forgetfulness, misunderstanding, guilt or ambivalence about sex, mood changes, or problems with side effects.

Noncompliance with the pill is very high: About 50 percent of teenagers stop taking it within a year of starting, even though they are still having sex (Ammerman). The reasons:

• Side effects, especially weight gain. Even a pound or two alarms some people, though medically it has no significance.

• Misunderstanding: A girl may be confused about the difference between disease prevention and pregnancy prevention. The pill works only for the latter. Or she may have heard that a friend got pregnant even though she was on the pill (an instance that is almost always human error).

• Confidentiality: A girl may be afraid that her parents will be told, that her compact will be discovered, or that a friend will tell her secret.

• Infrequent sexual activity: The pill involves a major change in the hormonal system — it may not seem worth the trouble for infrequent sexual activity. All methods involve some trouble, but using a condom probably makes more sense than going on the pill for protection which is needed only once a month.

• Self-esteem: Some girls feel ashamed or guilty because they are taking a contraceptive regularly — it's hard for some women to admit they are sexual beings. Sometimes women who are ambivalent have sex in order to get or hold a boyfriend. If a woman feels neglected or abused by her partner, she may lose her motivation to take the pill: She may either stop having sex, or try to get pregnant in order to get his attention.

If you find it difficult to take the pill as directed, for these or any other reasons, switch to another method of contraception that you will use consistently.

Frequently Asked Questions

What do I do if I forget to take a pill?

Ask your clinician when you get your first prescription. The answer depends on which pill you take. Generally, missing one pill can be remedied by taking it as soon as you remember. Then take the next pill at the regular time, even if it means taking two the same day. After that, it depends on the pill type. Ask in advance, or call for advice. Don't take chances: Use a back-up method of birth control until you are back on schedule.

If you forget to take your pills often, ask yourself: "Is this the right method for me?" It's an excellent method, but it's not the right choice for everyone.

Do I have to take the pill at the same time every day?

No, but you might want to. It keeps your hormone level constant, and you're more likely to remember to take it. Taking pills at different times can cause spotting or breakthrough bleeding. Many women take the pill when they get up in the morning. If you forget then, you still have all day to remember it. Others take it right before they go to sleep as part of their bedtime routine and because they are less likely to experience nausea if they are asleep. They can also check their packet in the morning to make sure they took it.

How much will the pill increase bust size?

Don't buy a new bra yet! If there is any change it is usually slight. Don't choose the pill for that reason.

Do Catholic women take the pill?

Yes. Many Catholics hoped that the oral contraceptive would be approved by the church, including Dr. John Rock, a leader in the development of the pill. But the church has not approved it, despite the fact that Catholics are just as likely as other couples to use birth control methods, and that the pill is one of the most popular.

I'm on the pill and didn't get my period this month. What should I do?

If you have not missed any pills and you miss one period without any signs of pregnancy, then pregnancy is very unlikely. Many women taking the pill occasionally miss a period. Call your health care provider if you're worried. If you forgot one or more pills and miss a period, stop taking the pill and use another method of birth control. Have a pregnancy test at your doctor's office. (Pregnancy tests in medical offices can detect pregnancy earlier than the urine tests from a drug store.)

When a woman wants to have a baby, can she count on getting pregnant after she stops taking the pill?

Yes. A woman who wants to get pregnant stops contraception at the end of a packet. Since it may be several months before she ovulates normally (her first non-pill periods may be irregular), it may be advisable to wait three to six months, using a non-hormonal method of birth control for that time, and tracking her periods to identify the fertile time (see Chapter 10).

Chapter 6

Diaphragm and Cervical Cap

You probably know the word diaphragm from the partition of muscle that separates the chest and abdomen inside the body. It lies under the lungs and heart and over the stomach, spleen, liver, pancreas and intestines. It moves when we breathe, sing, yell, or hiccup. "Dia"-"phragm" means "completely"-"enclose."

There is also a contraceptive called the diaphragm, so named because it encloses or covers a woman's cervix. The diaphragm is a "barrier" contraceptive in that—like condoms—it bars the way for sperm. It is very effective when properly used, which means *along with* spermicidal cream or jelly. Together, they provide a physical and chemical barrier between the sperm and egg. The cervical cap fits more tightly over the cervix; like the diaphragm it provides no protection against disease: These contraceptives do not cover the vaginal lining.

The diaphragm takes some practice to use—more than the condom, because it cannot be seen when it is in place. Most women who use the diaphragm are older, but many teenagers are satisfied with it as well. It can be put in place hours before intercourse, and if properly fitted it cannot be felt by either partner.

Carla, 16, got a diaphragm after deciding to go off the pill. "I had too many side effects from the pill," she said. "I was a little nervous when I first saw a diaphragm," she said. "I couldn't imagine how it would actually fit inside of me! But after the nurse showed me how to insert it and I practiced a few times, it was easy. I couldn't even feel it! And I like being able to put it in ahead of time so my boyfriend Alex and I don't have to worry about protection in the heat of the moment."

77

* * *

Jamie, 17, got a diaphragm after she and her boyfriend, Scott, started having sex. "I liked using the diaphragm, but I kept getting urinary tract infections," she explained. "My doctor told me it was probably from the diaphragm." Jamie now uses a cervical cap and says the urinary tract infections have stopped.

Since the diaphragm does not protect against STDs, a condom must be used as well, if there is any risk of infection. The two methods together virtually guarantees contraception (99+ percent protection against pregnancy) while protecting both partners against infection.

Diaphragm History and Background

The diaphragm is not a modern invention. The "original" primitive diaphragm or cervical cap might have been the shell of half a lemon (which the legendary lover Casanova recommended). It was inserted in the upper end of the vagina to cover the cervix, blocking the path that sperm travel to reach the egg. Other folk remedies resembling the diaphragm include leaves, gummy substances, seed pods, and wool.

The vaginal diaphragm was invented by a Dutch physician in about 1880. A dome of vulcanized rubber surrounded by a watch-spring, the device was used routinely in clinics for decades. It represented a major breakthrough for women, who then had some control over the occurrence of pregnancy. Margaret Sanger, who introduced the term "birth control," also popularized the diaphragm in this country. At one time, a third of all couples in the United States used it. By 1971 it had dropped in popularity, displaced by the pill and the IUD (intrauterine device). It still has a role, though, and many satisfied users.

How the Diaphragm Works

By itself, the diaphragm blocks passage of most sperm into the uterus. But that is not enough, since sperm can be active for five days after intercourse. Spermicidal (sperm-killing) cream or jelly must always be used with it, placed inside the dome or cup and around its rim. Then the rubber dome, with a flexible spring rim (arcing, coiled or flat), provides both physical and chemical barriers.

Spermicide is actually the more important part of the combination. As a barrier alone the diaphragm is not very effective. Its main job is to hold the spermicide in place. As with condoms, oil can damage rubber, so *never* use oil-based lubricants such as petroleum jelly with the diaphragm. If you need to use a lubricant during sex, water-based lubricants such as K-Y Jelly are fine.

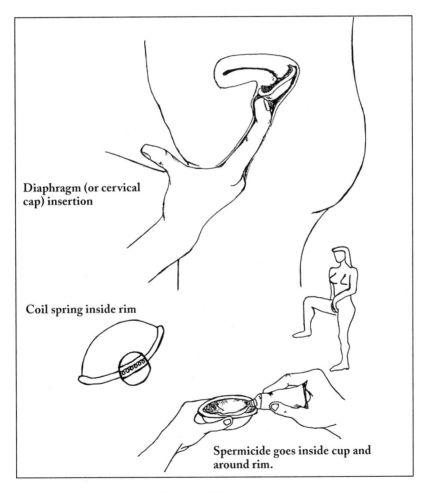

Diaphragm (or cervical cap) insertion

Coil spring inside rim

Spermicide goes inside cup and around rim.

Figure 5: Diaphragm.

Properly fitted and inserted, the diaphragm fits snugly over the cervix, sitting in place behind the pubic bone, and holding the spermicide toward the cervix. When you are first fitted for a diaphragm you will learn to put it in, check its position, and take it out. What is hard to describe in words or pictures will become clear with a little practice.

Women come in different sizes, and so do diaphragms. For a diaphragm to work right it must fit right, which is one reason why it requires a doctor's prescription. Diaphragms range in size from about two to four inches across, but are measured in millimeters (25.4 to the inch). The larger sizes are generally for women who have had several children and whose pelvic ligaments and vaginas have stretched; the smaller sizes fit teenagers and childless women.

Getting and Using the Diaphragm

To get a diaphragm, you must visit a doctor's office or clinic in order to be fitted. Spermicidal jelly and cream can be bought in any drugstore and in some supermarkets without a prescription.

Many factors affect a woman's satisfaction with the diaphragm as a method of contraception. One of the most important is how comfortable and confident you feel using it. Some women may be uncomfortable touching themselves and inserting the diaphragm inside their vaginas. A patient, understanding health care provider who can explain how the diaphragm should be used and who gives thorough instruction — including an opportunity for you to practice at his or her office — may help alleviate that discomfort. If you are simply not comfortable with such a method of birth control, by all means choose another. A good method used reluctantly is likely to be used sporadically, in which case it won't be very effective.

If you do choose a diaphragm, make sure you feel confident putting it in and taking it out before you leave your doctor's office and take it home. You wouldn't take a chance on diving into the swimming pool if your new bathing suit didn't fit right or you weren't sure how to fasten it closed. You would get used to it first by trying it on at home and moving around in it before putting it to the test in the neighborhood pool. The same idea applies to contraception. Get used to it before it's really needed. It's too late to learn in the heat of passion.

Julie wanted a diaphragm and was fitted by a well-qualified gynecologist who prefers other methods. He was not enthusiastic, and hurried through the explanation and demonstration. When she got home, Julie felt insecure about how to use it and, not surprisingly, was reluctant to try it with her boyfriend.

* * *

Jane got her diaphragm from a clinic that specializes in birth control. After a doctor had given her a pelvic exam and determined which size diaphragm she would need, a nurse showed Jane a life-sized model of the female pelvis with a diaphragm in place. Jane's cervix was no longer a mystery to her. The nurse explained how to insert the diaphragm, and Jane practiced alone, putting it in and taking it out a few times, then left it in for the nurse to check. Jane was sure of herself and very pleased with the diaphragm as a contraceptive method.

About a teaspoon of spermicidal cream or jelly is placed in the center of the dome, and a little is rubbed around the rim. The cream or jelly comes out of the tube like toothpaste; you should squeeze out about three inches' worth. Some women feel more secure if they also smear some spermicide on the outside of the diaphragm, too. But too much cream or jelly may cause the diaphragm to slip out of place, so don't overdo it.

Using the fingers of one hand, hold the rim of the diaphragm on either side and then pinch the sides together toward the middle. With the other hand, hold the labia slightly apart. It is best to do this in a sitting or squatting position, lying down with knees raised, or standing up with one leg up on a chair, edge of the bathtub, etc. The upper end of the diaphragm (the end nearest you) must be slipped far up into the vagina, up behind the cervix. When this is reached, the other end of the diaphragm is pushed up in front behind the pubic bone with your finger.

Use your finger to check the position of the diaphragm. You should be able to feel the tip of the cervix under the rubber. (The cervix feels like the tip of your nose.) If the diaphragm is in properly, you and your partner won't be able to tell it is there, except by manual examination.

You must put the diaphragm in within six hours before intercourse or genital contact. No matter when you insert the diaphragm, always use spermicide. If you put in the diaphragm more than two hours before having sex, you must insert a fresh supply of spermicide with the applicator before intercourse. The diaphragm *must* be left in place a minimum of six hours after the last act of intercourse. Do not leave the diaphragm in for more than 24 hours. During that 24 hours, fresh spermicide must be added each time you have sex. This is done using an applicator—the diaphragm remains in place the entire time. Fill the applicator with the cream or jelly and dispense it inside your vagina. An applicator usually comes with the cream or jelly. You can always get one when you get your diaphragm.

To remove the diaphragm, hook your finger under the rim and gently pull it out, allowing it to bend as it did when you put it in. After removal, wash the diaphragm with soap and warm water and carefully dry it with a towel. You may sprinkle it with cornstarch (but not talcum or perfumed powder—they can harm rubber). Keep it in its protective case away from heat. A diaphragm may become discolored over time, but you can still use it.

Check the diaphragm periodically for tears or holes by holding it up to the light or by filling it with water and seeing if any drops form on the underside. When well cared for, a diaphragm will last for a few years. It is a good idea, however, to get it checked at your yearly checkup and make sure it still fits well. You should also have it rechecked if:

- You feel it is slipping out of place.
- You have had pelvic surgery or have been pregnant.
- You have gained or lost a lot of weight.

Women who use the diaphragm should wear it whenever there is any possibility of intercourse. It is not uncomfortable, nor will it interfere with normal activities. If you're wearing it, you don't have to find the diaphragm, remember to put it in your bag, or say "Wait a minute— I've got to put in my diaphragm." As Naomi explained:

> "At first when I went out with my boyfriend I would just carry my diaphragm in my purse. But I could never find just the right moment to excuse myself to go put it in. Sometimes I'd wait to see if he would suggest I do it. Then I realized I could put it in ahead of time and not worry about it."

The only thing to remember about putting in your diaphragm ahead of time is to add more spermicidal cream or jelly with the applicator before intercourse if more than two hours have passed since insertion.

Even in those times when you end up putting the diaphragm in at the last minute, you'll find that, with practice, it takes only a few seconds.

Diaphragm Effectiveness

As with any birth control method, correct and consistent use of the diaphragm is key to protection. In typical use, the diaphragm has an 18 percent failure rate for a year of use. With perfect use, that failure rate is reduced to 6 percent.

Remember, the diaphragm *must* be used with a spermicidal cream or jelly. This means putting the cream or jelly in the diaphragm before inserting it and adding more with an applicator (do not remove the diaphragm) any time you have intercourse again within 24 hours. The spermicidal cream or jelly is just as important as the diaphragm itself in preventing pregnancy.

Remember, too, that the diaphragm must remain in place for at least six hours after the *last* act of intercourse.

Diaphragm Safety and Side Effects

For the majority of women, the diaphragm offers a safe, convenient method of birth control with no side effects. Some diaphragm users experience higher rates of urinary tract infections (UTI: infection of the bladder, urethra, or both). If you get a UTI, your doctor can give you antibiotics to treat it.

Women who have repeated UTIs should have the fit checked by a gynecologist. If it is right, they can try urinating soon after sex (and drink lots of water to keep the flow of urine high) and keep the diaphragm in no longer than eight hours at a time. But some women may need to switch to another method of birth control. In rare cases, a woman or her partner may be allergic to the latex rubber or the spermicidal cream or jelly.

The Diaphragm and STDs

The diaphragm does not protect against STDs. Use a condom with a diaphragm if there is any risk of exposure to infection. Spermicides are not germicides.

Conclusion

The diaphragm requires more practice than some other methods. Some women don't want to go to the trouble. But it offers benefits that many women appreciate.
- It is completely safe and has minimal side-effects.
- It is a local method. It affects only the part of the body where it is placed, not your body generally, like the pill.
- You only use it when you need it.
- It can be inserted ahead of time.
- Once you have learned how to use it, it takes only a few seconds to insert.
- It works well when properly used, and neither you nor your partner should even be aware of it.

Frequently Asked Questions About the Diaphragm

My diaphragm, which I've only been using for a few weeks, is changing color. Does that mean it's wearing out?
No. A diaphragm will change with use and exposure to air, from its original white color to a shade of beige or tan. This is perfectly normal and harmless.

My mother suggested that I get a diaphragm. She knows that my boyfriend and I have been having sex and explained to me that we had to take precautions. But I just can't bring myself to use it—I hate the idea of sticking it up inside myself.

Some women do not like the idea of touching their genitals or internal organs. There is a diaphragm inserter you can get (it's a short plastic stick), but you still have to check the position of the diaphragm and take it out by hand. You have two choices: Try to change your attitude and learn that there is nothing unclean or unhealthy about touching yourself, or choose another method of birth control. Choose a method of birth control that you like. Remember it only works if you use it.

Having intercourse several times and putting in more contraceptive jelly gets messy. What can I do?

Washing with soap and water between acts of lovemaking is fine. But *do not douche*, which will remove the spermicide. (We don't recommend douching in general because it is not necessary for normal feminine hygiene and can cause irritation and infection.) You might also try contraceptive cream instead of jelly. Creams are less lubricating and just as effective. Wiping the vulva with tissue or a clean, soft towel may also be helpful.

My boyfriend objects to the diaphragm. When we have oral sex before intercourse he says he can smell and taste the cream. I've tried different brands of spermicide.

It is best if both partners like a method of birth control. Have you tried washing the vulva with soap and water after putting in the diaphragm? This should remove any leaking spermicide. Once the diaphragm is in place, the jelly in the cup and around the rim should not spread down to the lower vagina before intercourse; it will be held against the cervix higher up. The problem is more likely to follow use of the applicator to add spermicide after the diaphragm is in place — try waiting a few minutes and then washing. If that doesn't help, switch to another method permanently or occasionally according to both your preferences.

I'm going to have an abortion; afterwards will I need a different size diaphragm?

Maybe. Bring it along and ask the doctor to advise you.

I find using the diaphragm very satisfactory, but I'm worried about its 18 percent failure rate. As I understand it, that means that after 100 women use it for one year, 18 of them will become pregnant. I've been using my diaphragm for a year, and I'm starting to worry that I might become part of those failure statistics.

Keep in mind that when the rates of failure for various birth control methods are compiled, it isn't always easy to distinguish between product failure and personal failure. No doubt, some of the failures in the statistics you cited resulted from improper use (or nonuse) of the diaphragm. Careful, correct use of a diaphragm plus a spermicide reduces the failure rate to 6 percent. And using the diaphragm for a year does not mean "your number is up." Each time you use it, you have the same 94 percent protection. You could, of course, switch to a birth control method that has a 99+ percent success rate: the pill, Depo-Provera or Norplant. If you want to keep using the diaphragm, you can increase your safety level by combining it with another method such as the condom (important if STD is a risk). Don't forget to add spermicide each time before you have intercourse.

Can you be fitted with a diaphragm if you've never had sex?

Yes. But it you may require a refitting after sex has begun, as the vaginal tissues stretch a bit (another good reason to start with condoms).

What if you start to menstruate while the diaphragm is in?

No problem. The initial flow usually is held in the cup of the diaphragm. But make sure you clean the diaphragm — as soon as it is safe to take out — in order to reduce the risk of toxic shock, a bacterial infection.

The Cervical Cap

A cervical cap is a small, flexible rubber cap that fits over the cervix and is used with a spermicide. It is similar to the diaphragm in that it provides both a physical and chemical barrier between the sperm and the egg. It is smaller than the diaphragm and it grips the cervix snugly, like a thimble on a finger. (The diaphragm is kept in place with pelvic structures.) Although it is somewhat more difficult than the diaphragm to insert and remove, it is more convenient in other ways: It requires less spermicide or jelly, it can be inserted a longer amount of time before intercourse, and it can be kept in for up to 48 hours.

Cervical Cap History and Background

The idea of the cervical cap is thousands of years old. In ancient Sumatra, women molded opium leaves into little cups to cover their cervixes. The cervical cap has been used in European countries for over a century, but was only approved by the U.S. Food and Drug Administration for contraceptive use in 1988.

How the Cervical Cap Works

Like other barrier methods, the cervical cap works to keep sperm out of the uterus. Like the diaphragm, it must be used with a spermicide. The cervical cap keeps sperm out by forming a tight seal around the cervical opening. The spermicide strengthens the seal between the cap and the cervix and kills any sperm that manage to get through the seal.

Getting and Using the Cervical Cap

Like the diaphragm, the cervical cap requires a prescription and must be fitted by a trained medical professional. Because not all practitioners are trained to fit caps, it's a good idea to call and check with them ahead of time. The cervical cap is available in four sizes, which means that many — but not all — women can be fitted with a cap. The cervical cap must be used with a small amount of spermicide, which is placed inside the cap before it is inserted into the vagina. The cervical cap is more difficult to fit because it is small and must fit over the cervix, which is up at the top of the vagina. A loose fitting cap will move and slip off.

Once you are fitted, your clinician will show you how to insert and remove it. Practice this several times before leaving the office. Make sure both you and your clinician check the cap to make sure it's fitted correctly. Take your time and get comfortable with handling the cap. As with anything, practice makes perfect.

Kelly and her boyfriend, John, had been using condoms for over a year and wanted to switch to a less "noticeable" method of contraception. At the clinic she visited, the doctor suggested she try the cervical cap. "I had never even heard of it before then," Kelly said. "At first I was afraid to try it — I thought, what if it gets stuck up there and I can't get out? How will I know if it's in the right place? But I practiced a lot at my appointment and got used to it. It's kind of like inserting a tampon without an applicator. John and I are really satisfied with it."

* * *

Deborah went to her gynecologist to get a cervical cap after her friend Jasmine recommended it. "I couldn't deal with it," she explained. "I guess Jasmine and I are different that way. I just couldn't stand having to touch myself down there so much, or reach up inside to check where it was. I knew I'd never use it, so I ended up going on the pill instead."

To use a cervical cap, fill it only one-third full of spermicide. Squeeze the rim of the cap and direct it into the vagina as far as it will go. Use your forefinger to press the rim around the cervix until the dome covers the cervix. Check for proper placement by sweeping your finger around the rim of the cap. Your cervix should be covered by the cap. After each act of intercourse, check the cap for proper placement over the cervix. Leave it in place for 8 to 12 hours, but not longer than 48 hours, after intercourse.

To remove the cap, push the rim to one side with your finger, then reach inside with the finger and gently pull it out (don't tear it with a fingernail). Wash it with mild soap and water after each use, dry it well and store it in its container. You can sprinkle the cap with cornstarch (but not talcum or perfumed powder — they can harm rubber). Keep it in its protective case away from heat. Check your cap frequently for holes by holding it up to the light or filling it with water and seeing if any droplets pass through. If cared for properly, the cap should last a few years.

When starting with the cap, use the condom or another method as a back-up for the first month or two. If the cap is consistently in place after sex, you can stop using the back-up method. But two methods are better than one: If the cap is ever dislodged, you will still be protected. (Consider two methods during your fertile days — see Chapter 10.) A cap that easily becomes dislodged needs to be refitted.

Although more difficult to use than the diaphragm, the cervical cap does offer some advantages: It can remain in place longer than the diaphragm (up to 48 hours), less spermicide is used, and you do not need to add spermicide before each act of intercourse. Also, many women find it less messy than a diaphragm, and urinary tract infections (UTIs) are less common than with the diaphragm because the cap does not press against the area next to the urethra. One disadvantage is that the cervical cap should not be worn during the menstrual period.

Cervical Cap Effectiveness

Failure rates for the cervical cap are the same as those for the diaphragm: 18 percent for average use and 9 percent for perfect use. But the failure rate is significantly higher for women who have given birth than for women who have not, perhaps because the cervical opening is wider after childbirth.

Checking for slippage will let a woman know if the fit is good.

Cervical Cap Safety and Side Effects

The cervical cap is a safe contraceptive method with minimal side effects. The most common problems associated with the cervical cap are vaginal odor and discharge, which are most likely to occur when the cervical cap is left in too long. If your cap develops an offensive odor, you may have a vaginal infection, so you should contact your health care provider.

It is also recommended that you have a Pap test and a cervical cap check after the first three months of use. The cervical cap may cause some cervical cellular changes, although more research on this is still being done. Women who have had an abnormal Pap smear should not use the cervical cap.

The Cervical Cap and STDs

Like the diaphragm, the cervical cap does not protect against STDs. A condom must be used with it if there is a risk of infection.

Conclusion

For many women, the cervical cap offers a convenient, effective method of contraception. However, it requires careful fitting by a trained professional and lots of practice by the user to make sure that it is inserted correctly and snugly in place. The effectiveness rates are significantly lower for women who have had children, so keep that in mind if you have already had a baby.

Frequently Asked Questions About the Cervical Cap

I'm worried about putting something so far up inside of me. Could it get lost in there?

No. The vagina stops about an inch beyond the cervix, so the cervical cap (or diaphragm or tampon, for that matter), cannot get lost. However, the cap can become dislodged during intercourse and you have to be diligent about checking it after lovemaking to ensure it is still in place. If you find that it is moving, you need to have the fitting checked by your health care provider.

Is the cervical cap uncomfortable?

If fitted and inserted correctly, neither you nor your partner should be aware that the cervical cap is there.

Chapter 7

Spermicides

All the methods we discuss in this chapter are based on chemicals that kill sperm. *Foams, creams, gels, films* and *suppositories* are different forms or types of *spermicide*. They are sold without need for a prescription at drug stores and supermarkets. A spermicide can be used alone, but its effectiveness in preventing pregnancy is much greater when it is used with a barrier method. Although foams were designed to be used alone, and are promoted as such, they are most effective when used with a diaphragm or condom. Creams and gels are meant to be used with a diaphragm or cervical cap; film (vaginal contraceptive film, or VCF) can be used with a diaphragm or condom; and a suppository — a waxy pellet that melts in the vagina — can be used with a condom.

Many other contraceptives are more effective than spermicides, but effectiveness is not the whole story. Convenience, cost, and access are also important. Some of the more effective methods — pill, Norplant, diaphragm — require a pelvic exam and a prescription. If you have hesitated to visit a health care provider, or have lost your diaphragm or missed a pill, you can always go to the drugstore for a can of contraceptive foam. It may not provide the best protection, but it's far better than no method, and it is improved if the male wears a condom.

History and Background

For a long, long time women have been using whatever they, their medical advisers, or "old wives tales" said would permit sex to occur without conception. Discussions of vaginal potions to prevent pregnancy are found in papyrus fragments written 4,000 years ago by Egyptian physicians. The Hebrew Talmud and the early Greek physician Soranus describe various techniques. Of course, the ancients had neither microscopes nor chemistry laboratories as we know them.

Our ancestors relied on theories beginning with guesswork and superstition, tested, if at all, by trial and error. Aristotle (384–322 B.C.), who greatly influenced both science and philosophy, suggested using oil of frankincense mixed with olive oil. Other early Greek sages advised peppermint juice mixed with honey. Also recommended were pomegranate pulp or rind, lemon juice, alcohol, alum, and cedar gum. Some of these recipes were on the right track — they could slow down, disable or kill sperm — but none can compare with what we have today.

How They Work

Spermicides contain an ingredient that kills sperm on contact. The chemical, most often nonoxynol-9, is carried in a base — cream, gel, film suppository or foam — that slows the movement of sperm. The active chemical in the spermicide disables and kills the sperm. The barrier effect is obviously not as good as a condom, diaphragm or cervical cap, and the chemical may not reach all the sperm.

Lila and Manuel had begun a sexual relationship the summer after their junior year of high school. Lila had been pregnant once before, with another boy, and had a miscarriage (spontaneous abortion). That pregnancy scare made her determined to take every precaution. They talked about what they would do as the romance developed over several months. They would be exclusive with each other — he would use condoms; she would use foam. It's working very well.

"We both are taking responsibility for the birth control, which I like. It doesn't just fall on one of us," said Lila. "There's something else that we like about the foam. Manuel has more of a sex drive than I do — probably like most guys, according to my girlfriends. We love each other so much, and I want to be close that way even at times when I can't get really aroused. He always can in a minute! He's patient and considerate but sometimes I'm not going to be lubricated enough by myself and the foam makes sex a lot more comfortable for both of us."

Manuel adds: "I like dry condoms better than lubricated — they're easier to put on. By using the foam we are more safe and everything goes real smooth!"

Getting and Using Them

These are all non-prescription, "over-the-counter" products. You can buy them at any pharmacy and most supermarkets; they are usually displayed with "personal products." Don't confuse contraceptives with feminine hygiene products like douches or plain lubricants, like K-Y Jelly. Some contraceptives are also lubricants, but lubricants alone won't give you any protection against pregnancy or disease.

Spermicides inserted vaginally remain effective for up to one hour. For foam, jellies and creams, contraceptive protection begins immediately after insertion. Film and suppositories require 10-15 minutes to melt and spread around before intercourse begins. For all spermicides, additional applications are required for each act of intercourse. A little may leak out, but it should not be washed out (douched). We don't recommend douching at all, but a woman who does so should wait six to eight hours after intercourse or she risks removing spermicide while leaving sperm in the vagina. Always read and follow instructions.

FOAM

Among spermicides, foam is the most effective when used alone. The foam has more "body" than cream or gel, provides a better barrier, and doesn't leak out, so it is less messy to use. Foams come in a pressurized can or vial from which you fill a clear plastic applicator or syringe. The first time you buy foam, make sure it comes with an applicator in the box. After that, you can buy foam refills and reuse the applicator from the first box.

Some brands of foam come with single doses inside disposable applicators. Others come in a can or plastic container, which you first shake well (20 times) and attach the applicator to the top. Push down enough to release the foam, and it will fill the applicator, pushing the plunger all the way out. Remove the filled applicator from the container.

Gently slide the applicator all the way up in the vagina (you may feel it touch the cervix). Then withdraw it slightly (about half an inch) so the foam can escape, and press the plunger all the way in. To make sure the foam goes where it should, high up near the cervix, it's a good idea to lie on your back when you insert it. Finally, remove the empty applicator, with the plunger all the way in, from the vagina.

Some women consider foam messy because it can liquefy and leak out. Also, because it must be introduced before each act of intercourse, spermicide might seem to lessen the spontaneity of lovemaking. Since careful and thoughtful lovemaking is always best — no unpleasant surprises later about "forgetting" contraception! — some lovers even make contraception part of foreplay. And once you've used foam, you'll find it's easy, quick and causes minimal interruption.

When the applicator fills very slowly and you hear a sputtering sound, it's time to get another container of foam. Keep an extra at hand to avoid either disappointment or unacceptable risk.

While not one of the most effective birth control methods, foam has its advantages. You can make it better in several ways:

• Use it with a barrier contraceptive — condom plus foam protects very well, as well as the pill. That also requires sharing the responsibility for birth control, which is good for your relationship, too.

• Use two full applicators instead of one.

• Insert additional foam if more than one hour has passed between the first insertion and intercourse.

• Insert foam before each act of intercourse.

• Deposit the foam in the upper vagina, not close to the vaginal opening. This gives proper protection and reduces leakage.

CREAMS AND GELS

These must be used with a diaphragm or cervical cap. Combined with barrier methods they provide excellent protection, alone they do not. Creams and gels (or "jellies") do not disperse evenly like foam. The diaphragm or cervical cap keeps the spermicide in place while it blocks passage of sperm into the uterus. Remember, there are hundreds of millions of sperm in each ejaculation, and it takes only one to fertilize an egg!

The process for using these chemicals is similar to that with foam. As with foam, we recommend that the male use a condom.) Fill the applicator by squeezing the spermicide tube. Insert the applicator into your vagina as far as it will comfortably go, pull it back half an inch, then push the plunger. A fresh application is required for each act of intercourse. Jellies and creams remain effective for up to one hour, but when used with a diaphragm or cervical cap (as they should be), they remain effective for 6 hours.

SUPPOSITORIES

Vaginal suppositories are made from a solid waxy material and do not need an applicator. This method wins over some women, who also like the fact that suppositories are less messy than other spermicides. Take off the wrapper and push the suppository up along the back wall of your vagina as far as you can so that it rests against or close to your cervix. Do this 10 or 15 minutes before intercourse so the suppository can dissolve and release the spermicide. But don't wait too long: No more than one hour can pass before sex is over, or the spermicide will be too weak. This takes some planning and the ability to adjust. If intercourse is not over within an hour, and you want to continue, then the male withdraws, you insert another suppository and wait another ten minutes before resuming intercourse. And, it's best if he uses a condom.

FILM

Vaginal contraceptive film (VCF) can be used alone, but is far more effective with a diaphragm or condom. Each film is 2" × 2" and paper-thin. Using her finger, a women inserts it on or near the cervix (or inside the diaphragm) about 15 minutes before intercourse to allow time for the film to melt and disperse the spermicide. (It might occur to you to put the film over the tip of the penis as a method of insertion, but the film may come off too far from the cervix and won't dissolve in time to do its work.) If more than an hour passes between insertion and intercourse, put another film in and wait another 15 minutes before resuming intercourse.

Store your spermicide supplies in a convenient place that is clean, cool and dark. After each use, wash the inserter with plain soap and warm water. Do *not* use talcum powder on it.

Effectiveness

To date, no studies have been done that compare the effectiveness of various types of spermicides. The National Institutes of Health (NIH) is starting one such study, with results expected in about four years. Other research indicates that, of 100 women who use foam, cream, gel, film or suppositories without another method, 21 will become pregnant during the first year of typical use. Only six will become pregnant with perfect use.

These are methods which leave a great deal up to the user. Couples should therefore use a condom (which also reduces disease risk) or other barrier method (diaphragm or cap, if neither partner is a carrier of STD) as well. But strict usage according to the directions — using spermicide with every act of intercourse; watching the clock for the right waiting times; and applying spermicides correctly — can make these methods up to 97 percent effective. Even the 21 percent pregnancy rate is about four times better than using no contraceptive at all: In a year of average frequency of intercourse, 85 percent of women will become pregnant if no method is used.

Spermicides can also be used as a backup option for a woman who is waiting to start oral contraceptives or for someone waiting for an IUD (intrauterine device) insertion. They also can be used as an emergency measure if a condom breaks. If that happens, an application of spermicide should be inserted immediately. Foam, cream or gel are better in that emergency because they dissolve faster than film or suppository. (See Chapter 12 for more about emergency contraception.)

Safety and Side Effects

Spermicides can be used by virtually all women. In rare instances, the spermicide may irritate the penis or vagina. Switching brands may solve this problem.

Some women (and men, too) are bothered by leaking of spermicide from the vagina; it feels messy. Couples who like to engage in oral sex sometimes find the taste of spermicides unpleasant (a small amount, even if swallowed, is harmless).

Spermicides and STDs

Studies indicate that nonoxynol-9 products might offer some protection against STDs such as gonorrhea and chlamydia. The risks for cervical cancer and for sexual transmission of hepatitis B virus also may be reduced. Remember, however, that abstinence, choosing a healthy partner, and latex condoms — in *that* order — offer the only real protection against STDs. Spermicides do not appear to protect against HIV. HIV/AIDS is a deadly disease, so spermicides alone should be used only if you and your partner are free of infection.

Conclusion

Spermicides are popular because they are easy to use, inexpensive, and are available over-the-counter. However, their effectiveness rates vary considerably because they are so dependent upon correct, consistent usage. They are much more effective when used in combination with another barrier method. Foam is the only spermicide to be used alone, and coupling it with a condom is much better. Gel, cream, film and suppositories should always be used with another barrier method.

Questions remain about how well spermicides protect against the spread of STDs. Don't take chances. Relying on spermicides alone for protection is like playing Russian roulette with two bullets in the chamber: one for pregnancy, one for disease. If there is any risk of exposure, either abstain from sex or use a condom with spermicide.

Frequently Asked Questions

Can you use any of the spermicides—foam, cream, gel or suppositories— with either a condom or a diaphragm or cervical cap? Or do you have to use foam with a condom, and cream or gel with a diaphragm or cervical cap?

Foam can be used by itself but is more effective in combination with a condom. The same is true for suppositories. Diaphragms and cervical caps require cream or gel to be effective, and cream or gel is only reliable when so used — not by itself. Spermicide improves the effectiveness of the condom and at the same time eliminates any problem of dryness.

Since you can get foam or cream without a prescription, they are what I tried at first. But by the time you insert it twice and then reinsert it, if you don't have intercourse immediately, it starts to feel too messy. What can we do about that?

A facial tissue or clean cloth takes care of this annoyance; leaked spermicide (at the opening of the vagina) serves no purpose, so it's fine to wipe it away. In the hours after lovemaking, if you're up and around, a sanitary pad can absorb any postcoital leaking.

What if, after inserting the foam, you have to urinate? Will this remove the foam or dilute it?

No. The opening of the urethra is outside the vagina, and the foam is high up inside. A bowel movement, however, might cause the foam to move down the vagina, so reapplication would then be advisable.

What if you feel burning or irritation, or some other allergic reaction to these products?

Very few people are allergic to these substances. However, ingredients do vary somewhat, and if you or your partner have any reaction, you can try another brand or switch to another birth control method.

Do spermicides protect me against STDs? What about HIV/AIDS?

Spermicides may provide some protection against chlamydia and gonorrhea, but they do not appear to protect against HIV/AIDS. If there is any risk of HIV infection, abstain from intercourse or use a latex condom with the spermicide.

Chapter 8

Norplant and Depo-Provera

Norplant and Depo-Provera are reversible methods of hormonal birth control that work like the pill, but on a long-term basis. They are injected or implanted under the skin, and are effective for months or years. The active ingredient is progestin, a hormone that stops ovulation and causes other temporary changes in a woman's body to prevent pregnancy.

Norplant is effective for five years after insertion, while each injection of Depo-Provera works for three months. These methods are good choices for women who have a hard time taking the pill, or who forget to take it. They are also better than the diaphragm for someone who "can't stop" in the heat of passion to put in her diaphragm. But these methods are not right for everyone. Many women have stopped using Norplant and Depo-Provera because they were not prepared for side effects, some of which are only mildly annoying and diminish with time. Others are more serious; knowing about them in advance prevents needless alarm. Abby, a high school senior, found Norplant worked well for her.

> "I didn't have to think about taking a pill every day and I knew I was using a very effective contraceptive. It seemed expensive when I first heard about it, but since it works for five years it's cheaper in the long run than buying pills every month."

Conversely,

> Naomi, 18, was not happy with her experience with Norplant: "I hated the side effects. It seemed like I had my period two

weeks every month, and I had lots of headaches and was tired. My doctor said to wait a few weeks and see if the side effects went away, but they didn't. So I had Norplant removed. I felt better after that."

Neither Norplant nor Depo-Provera contains estrogen, which makes them a good choice for women who do not tolerate products containing estrogen — the pill, for example (see Chapter 5).

Norplant was approved by the U.S. Food and Drug Administration in 1991, Depo-Provera in 1992. Both require a doctor's prescription and are administered by a health care professional. Although very effective in preventing pregnancy, they offer no protection against sexually transmitted diseases (STDs).

How They Work

Norplant and Depo-Provera prevent pregnancy hormonally, so ovulation does not occur.

For Norplant, six thin rubbery rods, about the size of match sticks, are inserted under the skin of a woman's upper arm. The implants release a hormone called levonorgestrel — similar to progesterone — which keeps the ovaries from releasing eggs. It also thickens the woman's cervical mucus, impeding transport of sperm into the uterus. It may also prevent a fertilized egg from attaching itself to the uterus.

Norplant prevents pregnancy for five years, and can be removed sooner than that if you choose. If you want to continue it beyond five years, a new set of implants is inserted in place of the first set.

For Depo-Provera, a synthetic hormone, medroxyprogesterone acetate, is injected into the buttock or arm. Each injection lasts for three months. The hormone prevents ovulation and also causes some temporary changes in the lining of the uterus that make pregnancy unlikely even if ovulation does occur. Some call it the birth control shot.

Getting and Using Them

Norplant and Depo-Provera require prescriptions, so you have to visit a doctor's office or clinic to obtain them. The doctor will examine you to make sure that Norplant or Depo-Provera are appropriate methods. Hormonal contraceptives — the pill, Depo-Provera, and Norplant — affect various parts of the body, so the physician has to consider any health conditions or risk factors you might have. If you are a good candidate for one of these, your clinician will explain how they work and discuss possible side effects.

For Norplant, a local anesthetic is injected first, and a small incision is made on the inside of the upper arm. Norplant capsules are inserted in a fan-shaped pattern. The area is bandaged, and no stitches are necessary. The procedure takes about ten minutes, and protection against pregnancy begins in 24 hours. (If you have sexual intercourse sooner than that, you must use another form of contraception.) The Norplant site may be sore for the first few days of healing.

Norplant is usually inserted within seven days of the start of your period: a precautionary measure to avoid starting it in a pregnant woman. Assuming you have no problems, there should be a follow-up visit in about three months to make sure everything is working well. After that, it is a good idea to have annual follow-up visits, unless there is a reason to have a checkup sooner. Norplant has to be replaced every five years. That is a long time in the life of a young woman, and if you use this method, you should have a fail-safe way to remember when you received the implant and when it "expires." You might carry a card in your wallet (coded to protect your privacy) or write in the date on a calendar.

To remove Norplant, your doctor numbs the same spot on your arm, makes a small incision, and removes the capsules. Because tissue forms around each implant, removal takes longer —15 to 30 minutes — and may cause more discomfort than insertion. It takes three to five days for the site to heal. If you want to continue using Norplant for longer than five years, you can get a new set of capsules at the same time the old set is removed. The new set can be put in the same arm as the first one, or in the other arm. Once Norplant is removed, its protective effect against pregnancy decreases rapidly, so it is important to begin using another method of contraception right away.

Depo-Provera is nicknamed "the shot" because it is injected by syringe and needle into the buttock or upper arm. To ensure you are not already pregnant, the injection is usually given during your period. Depo-Provera is effective immediately. An injection lasts three months, at which time you have to get another one, or change to a different method (if you are sexually active). Make sure you get your shot from a legitimate health care provider who is experienced with giving Depo-Provera. If you want to stop using Depo-Provera, simply avoid getting another injection.

Effectiveness

Norplant and Depo-Provera are extremely effective contraceptives. Of 10,000 women using Norplant for a year, only nine will become pregnant (.09 percent). In the case of Depo-Provera, of 1,000 women who use it, only three will become pregnant in the first year (.3 percent). One reason they are so effective is that it they are virtually error-free — there is no "human factor" such as putting in a diaphragm or taking the pill. Once Norplant is inserted, you don't have to do anything to prevent pregnancy for five years; with Depo-Provera you return to the clinic every three months. Compliance is automatic, and you don't have to remember to prepare for sex each time (barrier) or take something each day (pill).

But neither Norplant nor Depo-Provera provides protection against sexually transmitted diseases, so condoms must also be used if there is any risk of infection.

Safety and Side Effects

Many women use Norplant and Depo-Provera without difficulty, others have tolerable side effects, and some are unable to continue because of more bothersome side effects. For both methods, menstrual irregularities — ranging from longer periods to no periods at all — are the most common side effect. Some women like the lessening of menstrual flow and consider it an advantage of the method.

The most common reasons for discontinuing (removing) Norplant are irregular bleeding and weight gain. Irregular bleeding can mean varying intervals between periods, longer menstrual flow, bleeding or spotting between periods, or no bleeding for months (amenorrhea). Bleeding usually becomes more regular after 9 to 12 months. Weight gain is a common side effect with hormonal methods and is more problematic for some women than others. Less common side effects include acne, headaches, and depression. Any of these should be promptly reported to your health care provider. They may be treatable; but if not, you have to decide whether to tolerate the side effects or change methods.

Some women are deterred by the process of inserting the capsules. There may be scarring at the site of incision, although this is unusual. You also will be able to feel the capsules under the skin with your finger. Norplant is noticeable in some women, especially if they are lean or muscular.

Women who have liver disease, unexplained vaginal bleeding, breast cancer or blood clots should not use it. There are no statistics available yet on the risk of cancer associated with Norplant use. Many researchers expect the risk to be like that of using the pill — minimal.

Depo-Provera may not be right for you if you have liver disease, unexplained vaginal bleeding or a family history of breast cancer. As with Norplant, the most common side effect is irregular bleeding: longer or shorter intervals between periods, more or less menstrual flow, spotting between periods, or total absence of periods (amenorrhea). These changes are most likely to occur in the first 6 to 12 months of use. The longer a woman is using Depo-Provera, the more likely it is that her periods will stop. Over half of Depo-Provera users have no periods after one year, but periods and fertility usually return within 3 to 18 months after your last injection. But don't think that you're protected against pregnancy during that time — you're only protected if you've had a shot within three months. Other possible side effects of Depo-Provera include weight gain, headache, fatigue and mood changes.

Research has found that Depo-Provera may be associated with a decrease in the amount of minerals stored in bone tissue, possibly increasing the risk of bone fractures. Bone-mineral loss seems to be greatest in the early phase of Depo-Provera use, then it slows to the level of the normal age-related process. After Depo-Provera usage has stopped, bone density appears to return to normal. More studies are underway on this issue.

Women who use Depo-Provera have no increased overall risk of cancer of the breast, ovary, uterus, cervix or liver. But younger women (under 35) may have a slightly increased risk of breast cancer — about the same low risk as with the pill.

Depo-Provera is reversible, meaning that you should have no trouble getting pregnant after you stop getting injections. However, it usually takes longer for a woman who has used Depo-Provera to get pregnant than it does for a woman who has never used it. On average, it takes 10–18 months after your last injection to get pregnant. But this is a statistic which cannot be precisely predicted for any individual. After stopping any contraception, assume that you are immediately at risk for pregnancy if you are sexually active.

Norplant, Depo-Provera and STDs

Norplant and Depo-Provera do not protect against infection. In fact, the risk of infection may even be greater than usual when these hormonal methods are used, so you must use condoms if there is any chance of exposure to STDs.

Animal studies indicate that progesterone and related synthetic compounds, such as these two contraceptives, cause the lining of the vagina to become thinner. A thinner vaginal wall may be easier for viruses, including HIV, to penetrate. More research is underway to see if these findings apply to humans and whether women using these contraceptives are at increased risk for contracting STDs.

Conclusion

When Norplant and Depo-Provera became available in the United States in the early 1990s, people working on reproductive health issues were both excited and nervous. Many were encouraged by the high effectiveness rates of these methods in preventing pregnancy. However, some worried that some populations, such as teen mothers, might be pressured to use them since they were long-term methods — a form of temporary sterilization. These concerns were justified.

Shortly after Norplant was introduced in the United States, some elected officials, judges and others developed proposals for addressing issues such as child abuse, teenage pregnancy and welfare, that involved Norplant. For example, to stop child-abusing mothers from having more children, judges sometimes required them to use Norplant. Some state legislators who wanted to keep poor women (supported by welfare) from having more babies proposed laws with incentives to use Norplant, and penalties for having children. None of these laws passed, but they signal a disturbing trend.

It is easy to understand why some people make such proposals: Everybody wants to stop child abuse and reduce the number of children born into poverty. But these are drastic strategies that affect privacy and personal rights. They are not the best way to solve complex social issues. There is no evidence that such policies work, and they violate the Supreme Court's ruling that individuals have a fundamental right to control whether or not they will have children.

A related issue is the right of teenagers to accept or refuse long-term contraceptives. No state laws require parents to consent to their children getting contraceptives, including Norplant and Depo-Provera. Even so, some health care providers may refuse to give you Norplant or Depo-Provera unless you get your parents' permission. If that happens, decide whether you are comfortable involving your parents in this decision. If not, find another provider who does not require parental consent.

On the flip side is the situation where parents are concerned about their teenage daughter getting pregnant and ask a physician to give her Norplant or Depo-Provera. The parents want to know that their daughter is well protected from pregnancy if she has sex. But what if the girl wants to use another method, such as a diaphragm or the pill, instead? What should the physician do? What about the risk of STDs?

The American College of Obstetricians and Gynecologists Committee on Adolescent Health Care says: "The adolescent has the right to refuse any method of contraception and to discontinue contraceptives — which includes removal of contraceptive implants — without parental notification or consent." This is based on the adolescent's right to privacy and right to make reproductive decisions.

We agree that teenagers should have the final say in their own reproductive decision-making, including the kind of contraceptive they use. We also feel that avoiding premature childbearing is in the best interest of the adolescent, her family, future generations, and society in general. Sometimes trying to persuade someone to use a long-term method of contraception is all right, as long as the persuasion is done respectfully (without threats or coercion) and truthfully, so that the prospective user can give meaningful informed consent. That means educating a teenager about the importance of delaying childbearing until she's older and explaining how Norplant and Depo-Provera can help do that, along with comparing the two methods to other contraceptive options.

Norplant and Depo-Provera are ideal for many women, certainly for those who are sexually active but who cannot or will not use a method that requires repeated decisions and follow-through, and who do not experience serious side effects from hormonal methods. Yet, no one method is appropriate for everyone, and many teenagers are perfectly capable of using other methods consistently and effectively. Health care providers and family planning counselors should be able to promote the use of long-term contraceptives when appropriate, using the guidelines we have discussed, which are part of ethical medical and public health practice.

Frequently Asked Questions

I don't want to advertise that I'm on birth control. Will people be able to see the Norplant implants in my arm?

The implants are usually not visible. If you are very thin or muscular they may be noticeable. The skin over the implants may harden somewhat, and if you touch the site directly you can feel them. For these reasons, a woman who chooses Norplant should be aware that boyfriend, parent or friend might notice the implants.

I've read that it's really painful to get the implants put in and even worse to have them taken out. Is that true?

It can be, but not necessarily. To minimize discomfort, a local anesthetic is used to insert and remove Norplant. One way to minimize that risk is to find a health care provider who has a lot of experience with

Norplant. When you make an appointment, be sure to ask whether the doctor has been trained to use Norplant and whether he or she works with it frequently.

I can't decide whether to get Depo-Provera or Norplant. Both have things about them that I like and others that I don't. How can I decide?

First ask your health care provider; if he or she lacks experience with these methods, ask for a referral, or go to a family planning clinic that provides these methods regularly. Other sources of information include your local library, the Internet, or women's health organizations.

Depo-Provera might be a better choice for a woman who:
- Is concerned about even minor surgery
- Needs contraception for only a year or so
- Doesn't want anyone to know she's using contraception
- Doesn't mind injections

Norplant might be a better choice for a woman who:
- Wants a contraceptive that is good for up to five years
- Is very concerned about weight gain
- Doesn't want to have to get an injection every 3 months
- Is afraid of shots
- Is not concerned about minor surgery

Can the Norplant implants break inside my arm?

No. You should avoid putting direct pressure on the insertion area for the first few days, but after it has healed you can touch the skin over the implants. You can play sports. The implants won't break. You can ask your health care practitioner to show you the capsules before they are inserted. You'll see they feel like flexible plastic.

Will using a long-term method like Depo-Provera or Norplant interfere with my ability to get pregnant when I decide I'm ready?

No. Most women who stop using Depo-Provera can become pregnant within 10 to 18 months following the last injection. (Don't, however, take that to mean you're protected during those months after your last injection — protection decreases as soon as you stop getting shots.) Once Norplant is removed, you can become pregnant as easily as if you never used it.

Chapter 9

Intrauterine Device (IUD)

Available in the United States for more than 30 years now, the intrauterine device (IUD) was once so popular that ten percent of contracepting women used it. Today fewer than 500,000 women in the United States — 1.4 percent of those who use birth control — use one. Chances are you don't know anyone who uses an IUD for birth control. Why the drop in popularity?

In the 1970s, one type of IUD, the Dalkon Shield, was found to cause pelvic infections, miscarriages, and sterility. Thousands of its users reported these problems. Although it was taken off the market and newer, safer IUDs have been introduced, the "ghost" of the Dalkon Shield lingered on: Many people still believe that IUDs are dangerous. Actually, the IUDs now available are quite safe and effective. However, they are considered somewhat riskier with regard to infection, which sometimes leads to sterility, so they are not often recommended for women who are at risk for sexually transmitted diseases (STDs), or for those who want to have children later on (i.e., teenagers).

Because of its history, the IUD is treated as though it could contribute to infection and sterility. The evidence suggests that the device is better than its reputation. We present information on the IUD so that, with your own doctor, you can reach an informed and appropriate decision.

History and Background

Surprisingly, the IUD has an ancient history. Cleopatra (69–30 B.C.) — wife of her brother, Ptolemy XII, and mistress of Julius Caesar and Mark Antony — experimented with bits of dried sea sponge and other materials as primitive intrauterine devices. For centuries in the Middle East, camel drivers have known that pregnancy in a female camel is prevented by inserting pebbles into the uterus (important if the camel is needed for long trips across the desert). In the Middle Ages, some Persian women used uterine plugs of tightly bound paper tied with thread.

The trouble with such devices is that, when inserted under less than sterile conditions, they often lead to infection (the nature of bacterial infection was not known until the 19th century). Also, if the device is not inserted completely into the uterus, it can carry infections upward from the vagina, which is not completely sterile. The threads (or "tail") of the device, projecting down from the cervix, draw germs upward the way a candle wick draws wax.

With the exception of an IUD developed by Dr. Grafenberg in the 1920s, doctors never had success with this approach until the 1960s, when the modern IUD was introduced into the U.S. market. It became very popular, and millions of women had them inserted. They required no attention for years, they made no hormonal changes in a woman's body, they were very effective, and they didn't interfere with spontaneous sex.

Then in the 1970s it was reported that one IUD, the Dalkon Shield, was responsible for thousands of pelvic infections, miscarriages, infertility, and even several deaths. It was taken off the market, and use of IUDs fell dramatically. (Nearly 90 percent of IUD users are in their thirties and forties.) In the decades since, other IUDs have come onto the market. But even if women were not afraid of the earlier problems, doctors were. The Dalkon Shield was never approved by the U.S. Food and Drug Administration (FDA) and lawsuits resulting from its use led to a much more stringent review of all new contraceptive methods, including those currently on the market.

Only two IUDs are approved for use in the United States: the Copper T 380A (CuT 380A, or ParaGard) and Progestasert. The CuT 380A is by far the more widely used IUD and has been available in the United States for seven years. It is also the only IUD that can be used as an emergency contraceptive (see Chapter 12).

How It Works

The CuT 380A is made of plastic and copper molded into a T-shape, with two plastic threads tied to the bottom. It is inserted into the uterus by a trained health professional, where it can remain for up to 10 years. Progestasert contains no copper and is generally only prescribed for women who cannot use the CuT 380A for health reasons, such as an allergy to copper. It is hormone-releasing and must be replaced annually.

Despite years of study, we still don't know exactly how the IUD works to prevent pregnancy. Until recently, researchers believed it prevented fertilized eggs from implanting themselves in the womb. More recent studies indicate that the IUD causes a harmless inflammation of the uterine lining, which disrupts the movement of the sperm and makes it difficult for it to reach and fertilize the egg. The inflammation subsides after the IUD is removed.

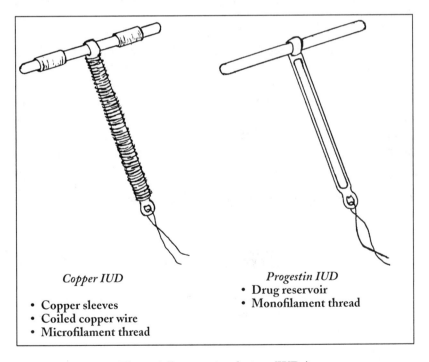

Copper IUD

- Copper sleeves
- Coiled copper wire
- Microfilament thread

Progestin IUD
- Drug reservoir
- Monofilament thread

Figure 6: Intrauterine devices (IUDs).

Getting and Using It

The IUD must be inserted and removed by a trained health professional. In a 15-minute procedure in the doctor's office, the cervix is slightly dilated (widened) and the IUD is inserted into the uterine cavity under sterile precautions.

Some women experience pain during insertion, but it is usually brief and feels like bad menstrual cramps. Women who have not had children (nulliparous) are more likely to have pain or cramping during insertion than women who have had children (parous). Pain medication can help, and antibiotics may be given to reduce the chance of infection when the IUD is inserted.

A string on the IUD hangs down through the cervix into the vagina. You should feel for the string from time to time, especially after menstruation, to make sure the IUD is still in place. If you can't feel the string, or otherwise suspect the IUD is not in place, call your health care provider and use another form of birth control in the meantime. You will need to have a checkup three months after insertion, and annually thereafter. The CuT 380A can be left in place for up to ten years, at which time it can be replaced, while the Progestasert must be replaced annually.

Despite the low usage rates for IUDs, those who choose it tend to stick with it. Approximately 81 percent continue to use the device after the first year, a much higher percentage than for other methods such as the pill or the diaphragm. Not all health care providers insert IUDs. If yours doesn't, try a local family planning clinic for an appointment or referral. The cost ranges from $150 to $300. While this may seem expensive, it pays for up to a decade of protection. The IUD can only be removed by a trained health care provider.

Effectiveness

The IUD is one of the most effective methods of birth control available to women in the United States. With typical use, the first-year failure rate is 0.8 percent for the CuT 380A and 2 percent for the Progestasert. With perfect use, it is 0.6 percent for the CuT 380A and 1.5 percent for Progestasert.

Safety and Side Effects

The legacy of the Dalkon Shield has lingered, and many people — health care providers and women alike — still mistakenly believe that the latest IUDs pose the same risks as the Dalkon Shield. This is not true. In fact, at a government-sponsored 1996 conference on IUDs, public health officials and researchers agreed that IUDs are effective and safe for women who are not at risk for STDs.

However, a woman who has an STD and uses an IUD is at much greater risk for contracting pelvic inflammatory disease (PID), which can lead to sterility. This is why a woman who uses the device must have only one sex partner who is also monogamous. Women who have not had children are not ideal candidates for the IUD: Although infection is rare, its occurrence might lead to sterility. Also, women who have had unexplained abnormal vaginal bleeding, a recent history of pelvic infection, a history of tubal pregnancy, or a recent abnormal Pap test should not use an IUD.

Possible side effects from an IUD include cramping (either after insertion, during periods, or both); bleeding between periods; heavier, longer periods; slightly increased risk of PID; and a small risk of uterus perforation during insertion. There is a small chance that the IUD could fall out; and if you aren't aware of that, pregnancy could occur. Pregnancy with an IUD in place is rare, but if you do get pregnant it is important that the IUD be removed as soon as possible to protect you and the fetus.

The IUD and STDs

There is no protection against STDs from an IUD. In fact, it may make infection more likely and more serious, causing pelvic inflammatory disease and leading to sterility. Unless you are in a mutually monogamous relationship, the IUD is not a good choice.

Conclusion

The IUD is best for a woman with one partner, where both are free of disease and have an exclusive sexual relationship with each other; and the woman should already have all the children she wants. It is a long-term contraceptive (up to 10 years) and is completely reversible, relatively economical, and low-maintenance (just check the string periodically). Women who are at risk for STDs (those with multiple partners, for example) should not use the IUD. Women who have not completed their childbearing should be very cautious about using the IUD for the reasons indicated.

Frequently Asked Questions

Is it true that an IUD has to be inserted during menstruation?
An IUD can be inserted any time during the cycle as long as you can be sure you're not pregnant. The advantage of inserting it during your period is that it ensures that you're not pregnant; also, the cervix is already slightly open at that time.

Even if I don't want to use an IUD as my ongoing contraceptive method, can I use it as an emergency contraceptive?
Yes. The CuT 380A can be used as an emergency contraceptive, and it is an effective one. It must be inserted five to seven days after unprotected sexual intercourse and can be removed after pregnancy is no longer a possibility, or it can be left in as a woman's ongoing method of contraception. (See Chapter 12.)

If I can feel the strings of the IUD coming down from the cervix, will my boyfriend be able to feel them during sex?
Very unlikely. The penis is sensitive, but not the way a fingertip is.

Chapter 10

Natural Family Planning (NFP)

Understanding the menstrual cycle is important, even though the natural family planning (NFP) method by itself is not one of the most effective. It's called "natural" because there is nothing to insert or put on, no pill to take. NFP only requires a woman to identify the bodily signs and symptoms of fertility — the time of the month she can become pregnant. She and her partner can then choose the timing of sexual intercourse to avoid the fertile time of the month if they wish to decrease the chances of pregnancy. The "safer" days are those when she is unlikely to get pregnant.

The method is not easy because a woman needs to know her reproductive cycle well and track it carefully. NFP is sometimes referred to as "fertility awareness" or "periodic abstinence" since you must abstain from sex during the "unsafe" (fertile) days. June, a college freshman, said,

> "I like natural family planning because you don't need prescriptions. All you need is a knowledge of how your body works, and regular periods. I would never use it if my periods weren't regular, though. Then it's like playing Russian roulette!"

There are three techniques for figuring out when your fertile time occurs: *the rhythm method, the basal body temperature method, and the cervical mucus method.* A combination of these three is called the *symptothermal* method and is more effective than each used alone. Another method, the *postovulation method*, involves abstaining from sex from the beginning of your period until the morning of the fourth day after your predicted ovulation, more than half your cycle.

Natural family planning is not an exact science. This type of family planning has a failure rate of 14 to 20 percent: After a year of average use, about 17 out of 100 women will become pregnant. With perfect use, the symptothermal method claims a better rate—only 2 percent failures. But for women who have irregular cycles, "perfect use" is not likely to be attained.

While it is less effective than other methods, NFP is far better than nothing. It can be used to make other methods better. And, used alone, it is the only method of birth control approved by the Catholic church. Since the method is based on fertility awareness, women who want to have children can use their knowledge when they are ready to become pregnant.

It should be obvious that these methods provide no protection against sexually transmitted diseases (STDs).

History and Background

Scientific understanding of the timing of ovulation dates back to about 1930—relatively recently. Before that, assumptions about the likeliest time to get pregnant were guesswork and varied widely.

The rhythm method, the basal body temperature method, and the cervical mucus method are all strategies for figuring out exactly when you ovulate—that is, when the egg is released from the ovary. Pregnancy results from the union of sperm and egg. Like other methods, NFP helps prevent that union while permitting sexual relations.

Estimates of the number of fertile days per menstrual cycle have ranged from two to ten, based on the survival of sperm and eggs. Data from an excellent new study indicate that the fertile period is six days, ending on the day of ovulation (Wilcox et al. 1995). The egg is only viable for a day, while sperm can survive for up to five days in the female reproductive tract.

It is difficult to figure out exactly when you are going to ovulate. You must keep a careful record of many monthly cycles in order to find the interval (most probable day) for ovulation, counting from the first day of your most recent menstrual period. Besides counting days, there are other ways to help pin down the time an egg is released. You can also take your temperature and check the vaginal mucus, as described below.

How It Works

RHYTHM

Many girls have heard of rhythm, and many even think they are using it. But they are often unsure about what time of the month is safer, and what time is fertile. The usual fertile time is midway between periods. *The safest time starts after ovulation and lasts until the next menstrual period.*

The rhythm, or calendar, method requires you to chart your menstrual cycles on a calendar. If you have very regular cycles, every 28 days, then you can expect to ovulate about day 14. You abstain from intercourse for six days: five days before, plus the day of ovulation. Abstaining longer is safer, since you might ovulate early one month. To calculate your safe period, start by keeping a written record of your menstrual cycles. You need eight to twelve cycles for reliable calculations. Count from the first day of one period until the day before the next period begins, then start a new count.

Theoretically, if sex were avoided for six days—five days before ovulation and 24 hours following it—pregnancy would not occur. Six days' abstinence in a typical cycle of 28 days still allows intercourse for three out of four weeks. The question is, how do you know which six days are fertile, or "unsafe"?

1 _ _ _ _ _ 7 _ x x x x x x (14) _ _ _ _ _ _ 21 _ _ _ _ _ _ 28

Using the four week calendar above, take day one as the beginning of menses (menstrual flow). It begins 14 days after ovulation. In a regular 28-day cycle, ovulation occurs on day 14, and the six fertile days will be 9–14 (marked with "x").

If an egg is not fertilized, it dies. The built-up lining of the uterus (endometrium) disintegrates and is expelled vaginally. This is the menstrual flow. In the example above, the next menses would begin after day 28, or day one of the next cycle.

Marilyn is a young woman who has irregular cycles. She kept track of twelve cycles; the longest was 32 days and the shortest was 26 days. To use NFP effectively she should abstain from day 8 to day 19 (12 days) since the day of ovulation can vary from day 13 to day 19. Using techniques to be described below, she can detect the day of ovulation and know that her fertile days are over until the next cycle begins. In order to be even safer, she can abstain longer — from day one until ovulation: Even after tracking 12 cycles she might ovulate even earlier or later than expected.

Use the shortest cycle to find the first day in your cycle that you are likely to be fertile. Use the longest cycle to find the last day you are likely to be fertile. Because many teenage girls have irregular periods, some may have to abstain more than half the time each month. Calendars to help you keep track are available from Catholic and other family planning clinics, gynecologists, and women's health centers.

Basal Body Temperature (BBT)

The calendar method can be supplemented with the use of a special thermometer to determine the time of ovulation. As a result of hormonal activity at the time of ovulation, the release of the egg coincides with a slight change in a woman's body temperature. To detect this change you need a basal thermometer that measures tenths of a degree. Most basal thermometers can be used orally, rectally or vaginally: Oral is easier, while rectal and vaginal are more accurate. Whichever you choose, use it consistently. Basal thermometers can be purchased at drug stores and usually come with instructions and a temperature chart.

To learn what slight signal your own body sends out when ovulation occurs, you must take your temperature each morning at the same time before getting out of bed. Any kind of activity can throw the reading off, so you cannot go to the bathroom, eat something, or make a phone call before taking your temperature. Suppose you find that your resting morning (basal) temperature is usually 97.7 degrees (usually it is a little lower in the morning than later in the day). *Just before ovulation your temperature should drop about three-tenths (0.3) of a degree*, to about 97.4. Then, *when you ovulate, your temperature will rise about five or six tenths (0.5 or 0.6) of a degree* above your normal, to about 98.3.

If the egg is not fertilized, it will disintegrate within three days, during which time the temperature remains at least 0.5 degrees above the basal level. The average temperature in the second half of the cycle is usually slightly higher than in the first, but your temperature should drop toward basal level after a few days if you are not pregnant. (Note:

If you are sick and running a fever, this will throw off your calculations.)

The calendar and thermometer complement each other and provide you with important information about your cycle. The thermometer helps provide a check on your calendar calculation of ovulation and fertile days. It will let you know about an early or late ovulation. The problem is that the information may come too late, if you already have had intercourse on a fertile day and didn't realize it.

CERVICAL MUCUS

Another supplement to the calendar, this technique involves observing changes in your cervical mucus for clues about when you are fertile. Normally, the mucus is cloudy and tacky, like cottage cheese, but a few days before ovulation it will become clear and slippery, stretching between the fingers like raw egg white, and there will be more of it. When this happens, a woman is fertile and must refrain from sexual intercourse to avoid pregnancy.

To get used to the mucus changes in your cycle, it is a good idea to record them for a few cycles. Keep in mind that semen, contraceptive foam, diaphragm jelly or lubricant can interfere with your ability to detect a mucus pattern. Also, the amount of discharge varies throughout the month, and some women may not be able to detect any at certain times. To get to know your own pattern, check the mucus each day whenever you go to the bathroom by wiping the outside of your vagina with toilet tissue from front to back. Feel the mucus and record the wettest mucus noted for each day.

Using It

Few teenagers use NFP. While other methods of birth control require you to anticipate first intercourse by only a matter of days or weeks, with NFP you must anticipate first intercourse by up to a year while you record your menstrual periods. Some teenagers already record periods on a calendar to keep track of them, which may make the rhythm method easier for them. Despite its relatively high failure rate, some young women do use NFP.

Marcia, 17, explained, "When my older sister was engaged to be married, she got the chart and some other things from a Pre-Cana conference, or maybe from her doctor. Anyway, I asked her what all that stuff was, and she explained the rhythm method. Knowing about it, I figured I'd just start keeping my own chart."

* * *

Edith, 19, said, "Using rhythm means that my boyfriend and I have only about ten safe days a month. That keeps sex a special occasion — we don't take sex for granted in our relationship; we don't treat it casually and so we appreciate it more."

Some girls simply operate on the principle that the middle of the month is "unsafe" and have sex at times close to their period. Luck and the law of averages will keep some of them from becoming pregnant, but not all.

For couples who use other methods and want to improve their effectiveness, using rhythm can be very helpful as an extra form of security. If you use the pill properly, there is no need to use rhythm, since there is no ovulation. But since the diaphragm, condom and foam can sometimes fail, knowledge of your unsafe days is a good supplement to these methods. If you are using either foam or the condom, you can calculate the fertile days and use both together at that time. There are no statistics on the effectiveness of this combination of three methods (NFP, condom and foam), but it is likely near 100 percent.

Effectiveness

The effectiveness of the rhythm, cervical mucus and basal temperature methods depends upon the user. Experts suspect that sexual risk-taking during fertile days accounts for more accidental pregnancies than does failure to interpret charts accurately. Among typical users of fertility awareness, approximately 20 percent will become pregnant during the first year. Among perfect users, the failure rate is ten percent or less.

Percent of Women Experiencing an Accidental Pregnancy
Within the First Year of NFP
[Adapted from Hatcher et al., 1994]

Method	Typical Use	Perfect Use
Chance	85	85
Fertility Awareness	20	
Calendar (Rhythm)		9
Ovulation method (Cervical mucus)		3
Symptothermal (Rhythm, cervical mucus and temperature)		2
Postovulation		1

Natural Family Planning and STDs

With regard to sexually transmitted diseases, there is *no safe time* of the month. Temperature, cervical mucus and menstrual cycle tell you nothing about your risk of contracting an STD. Any time you have sex without a latex condom, you are at risk for contracting an STD such as chlamydia, gonorrhea and HIV. Unless you are in a monogamous relationship with someone you know is disease-free, NFP is high-risk unless you combine it with a latex condom. Then you'll get double the protection — against pregnancy and STDs.

Conclusion

Natural family planning is relatively inexpensive, has no dangers or side effects, and is the only family planning method endorsed by the Catholic church. The basal thermometer and charts for tracking your cycle are relatively inexpensive. Slide rules, special calendars and other special aids that are available to help improve your use of NFP methods aren't necessary. You can make your own calendar-chart, and the Internet has many examples available (see Resources Appendix).

Natural family planning requires a great deal of dedication. If it is all you can do, do it right. That means using all three techniques together: rhythm, cervical mucus and basal temperature — and using them diligently. Women who rely only on NFP are likely to have some missteps in their reproductive years. It's good to understand rhythm and how your body works, but NFP works best as a supplement to other contraceptive practices, especially for young women who are not yet ready to have children. And because this method provides no protection against STDs, it should only be used by women who are in monogamous relationships with partners they know are disease-free.

Frequently Asked Questions

If rhythm has such a high failure rate, why does anyone want to use it?
Many Catholics consider it their only choice besides total abstinence if they do not wish to have a baby. Also, rhythm does not require a woman to go out and get a contraceptive method. Girls who are embarrassed or afraid to visit a family planning clinic may feel it is better than nothing — which it is (17 pregnancies per 100 woman-years, versus 85 for no method).

Are there some women who shouldn't try to use rhythm?
About 15 percent of women have such irregular cycles that they cannot rely on the rhythm method. It would not suit a girl whose cycles vary by more than 10 days.

Can I use an ovulation predictor kit to help me figure out the safe and unsafe times during my cycle?
No. Ovulation predictor kits, which are available without a prescription at most drug stores, are not intended to be used as contraception. They are for women who are trying to become pregnant and want to find out when they are most likely to be fertile. Given that your fertile period *ends* with ovulation, the predictor kits are entirely useless as a contraceptive aid.

Is it dangerous to have intercourse during the menstrual cycle?
No. Some couples refrain because they find it less pleasant. In some cultures the menstruating woman is "taboo." But menstrual blood is not

unsanitary. If a woman's flow is light and she has no cramps, she may enjoy sex during her period, in part because of the increased desire some women feel at this time and in part because it is the safer time from the standpoint of pregnancy risk.

Is there any reason to record my menstrual cycle if I'm not using NFP?

We recommend that all women, whether or not they use NFP, chart their cycles in order to get to know their own patterns. You may observe headaches, mood swings, and other changes that go along with regular hormonal fluctuations.

Chapter 11

Other Methods—and Some "Nonmethods"

The good news is that you have a choice of several excellent contraceptive methods. The bad news is that no one method is perfect, and what is best for one person will not suit everyone. You don't need to know all about every method, just the main things about a few methods, so you can weigh and discuss the pros and cons with your partner.

Most people can find at least one method that is both effective and convenient. The choice depends upon your personal needs and experience. Things change: What is right for you at one time may not be the best choice later on. The condom, for example, is the best first method for most people, but a couple in a long-term relationship and with no risk for STD may prefer the diaphragm or the pill.

You can drive a car without knowing how the engine works, and you can rely on expert mechanics if trouble develops. When it comes to sex, the more you know the better, because going to an expert is not quite as easy as pulling into a gas station, and the questions are too personal to ask just anyone. The more you know about your body and about birth control, the happier you will be with your choices about sex and family planning. The Scout motto "Be prepared!" applies here (though it was not intended for this). Knowledge is power, and knowing your options pays off in terms of less worry and better outcomes.

In this chapter we talk about methods that are either less reliable, like withdrawal, or that are not used by young people, like sterilization. We also talk about "nonmethods," things people do to prevent pregnancy—like douching—that don't work. Finally, we talk about future birth control methods.

Other Methods

WITHDRAWAL

The Latin term is *coitus interruptus*, interrupted sexual intercourse. With this technique the male tries to prevent sperm from entering the vagina during intercourse by withdrawing his penis (pulling out) just before his climax (ejaculation). This is an old practice, mentioned in the Bible as the sin of Onan. It reduces the chance of pregnancy, but there are two problems. First, ejaculation accompanies a pleasurable feeling of loss of control. Not many men — especially younger men — can tell exactly when the climax will occur. When they do know, it is too late to stop, and the strong desire is to thrust inward, not pull out. The second problem with the method is that it provides no protection against STD. In HIV-infected men, infected cells may be present in drops of fluid coming from the penis *before* climax. Even withdrawing at ejaculation may be too late to prevent HIV transmission. The withdrawal method has a typical failure rate of 19 per 100 (the pill is less than 5 per 100). It is better than no method, but there are lots of better methods available.

Sperm are very effective in reaching the egg, if one is present. There are cases in which a virgin became pregnant because her boyfriend ejaculated on the vulva during nude petting without intercourse. Sperm entered the small virginal opening in the hymen, traveled up the vagina into the womb and reached the egg in the Fallopian tube.

Withdrawal has a long history. In the nineteenth century the French birth rate fell, perhaps because of the widespread practice of withdrawal at a time when smaller families had advantages.

Nowadays only two percent of sexually active women report relying solely on withdrawal, but many men have probably used this method at some time in their lives. Why? Withdrawal costs no money and requires no advance planning. It's always available in the "heat of the moment." But keep in mind that you get what you pay for: some protection and a lot of anxiety. Sex is never an emergency, but its power draws people to the edge of disaster and many go over.

Some men develop great skill in controlling sexual arousal and climax. They can use withdrawal more effectively. But most young people cannot practice withdrawal with any reasonable hope of success. Sex is new, urges are strong, control is weak. Accidents happen. Be wary of a guy who boasts about his ability to control himself. It may be true, but if it's not you may find out the hard way. Some guys lie in order to have sex, and even so they won't have to bother with a condom: "I'll pull out in time" is a promise we would not bet much on.

Besides the consequences of pregnancy and disease, withdrawal has psychological risks. The partners have to interrupt their pleasure, their closeness, at the height of passion. They have to break off lovemaking at the worst possible moment. And they have to worry about that when they should be relaxed. Anxiety often ruins sex, especially for the woman. She bears more of the consequences, and her sexual enjoyment depends on being free from fear. Just a little more knowledge and preparation make intimacy with the right person a time of celebration — the best reason for postponing sex until you are really sure.

STERILIZATION

Vasectomy and tubal ligation for male and female, respectively, are safe, effective and permanent forms of birth control used mainly by people in their mid-thirties or older who have had all the children they want. We discuss it here so you will understand it, not because you will use it any time soon. Sterilization is permanent because it is hard if not impossible to reverse. It is not for young adults who may want to have children, but it is a blessing for couples who have finished childbearing because they need no longer bother with any contraception. Assuming that the partners are free of disease and faithful to each other, only one partner needs the operation.

Let's define some terms. "Sterilize" has two different meanings here. One refers to germs and infection: We sterilize a baby's bottle by boiling, and surgical instruments are sterilized with heat or chemicals before an operation to prevent infection. The second meaning has to do with sperm and egg, which are not germs in the usual sense, but germ cells, meaning they can grow unlike any other cells in the body. Men and women are "fertile" if they provide healthy sperm and eggs, respectively. If the words remind you of farming, that's fine: We fertilize crops so they'll grow, we sterilize (geld, spay) animals so they won't reproduce.

Here *infertility*, or *sterility*, means the inability to have a child (and offspring and crops, if we include animals and vegetables). Sterilization—permanent birth control—stops reproduction and brings about infertility. It has nothing to do with *potency*, which is the man's ability to have an erection and climax during sexual intercourse. It also has nothing to do with castration, which means removal of the gonads (testis or ovary; but "castration anxiety" in psychology refers to loss of the penis). Vasectomy and tubal ligation leave the gonads intact while blocking (tying off) the passageways for egg and sperm. The gonads produce hormones (testosterone, estrogen) which make adult males and females different; these hormones go directly into the blood stream and do not pass through the spermatic duct or Fallopian tubes.

Male castration refers to removal of the testicles, not the penis. Psychoanalyst Sigmund Freud introduced the term "penis envy," which referred to the confusion and curiosity of young children about the differences between the sexes. "No, you can't touch my penis," says the little boy to his sister, "you already broke yours off!"

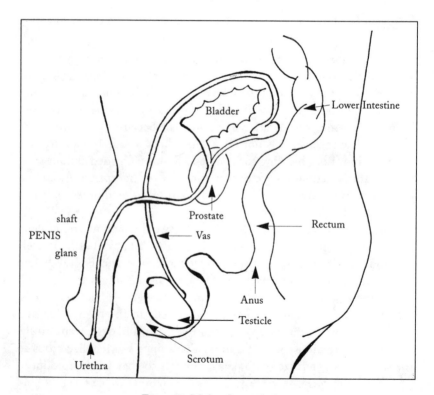

Figure 7: Male—Lateral view.

The male sterilization operation is called vasectomy. (*Vas*, Latin for "vessel"; *ec*, "out"; *tomy*, "cut.") The method consists of tying and cutting a tiny tube (as thin as angel hair pasta, called *vas deferens*, or *spermatic duct*) on each side of the scrotum. Sperm are still made but no longer travel from testes to urethra; instead, they are just absorbed. Seminal fluid, mostly from the prostate gland, comes out normally with orgasm. Since sperm are less than five percent of the ejaculate, you can't tell any difference after vasectomy without a microscope. The vasectomy procedure, minor surgery, takes about 20 minutes in a clinic or doctor's office.

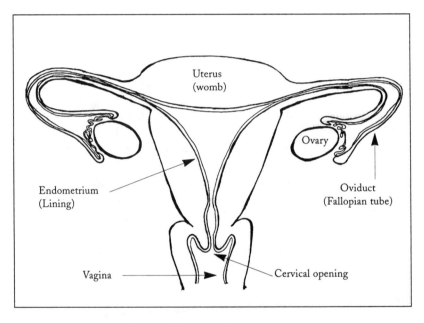

Figure 8: Female—Anterior view.

Tubal ligation in the female seals off both *Fallopian tubes* (also called *oviducts*, they are about spaghetti-size). Eggs can no longer meet sperm and proceed into the uterus. Tubal ligation used to be major surgery, but nowadays a mini-laparotomy, under local anesthesia, can be done through a small incision in the abdomen. This is a low-risk procedure but still more complicated than vasectomy, since the woman's tubes are inside the body while the man's are in the scrotum, which is a kind of outside pocket.

Female sterilization is the single most popular birth control method in the United States today: Women whose childbearing is over are glad to have a safe, permanent method. Surprisingly, however, it is not perfect. Over a ten-year period, about one in 50 women got pregnant, according to a recent study. Evidently a tube can grow back together after it is cut and the two ends are tied off. The younger the woman at the time of sterilization, the higher her risk of getting pregnant. No comparable long-term studies have been done on vasectomies, but researchers believe they are more effective. It is estimated that one in 1,000 vasectomies fail on the first year. Nothing is perfect, but vasectomy and tubal ligation are among the most effective birth control methods for older couples.

Combination Methods

If one is good, are two methods better? Yes, almost always. As we have suggested in the earlier chapters, the less effective methods ought to be combined for best results. Here we review and summarize such combinations.

The condom should always be used in a new relationship because of the possibility of disease, even if a woman is already using the pill or IUD. Less effective methods, such as the diaphragm, can be coupled with timing (rhythm or NFP) or condoms. Vaginal foam is a good second method to back up others (except the diaphragm). If foam is your basic method, it should be supplemented during the fertile days with a condom or abstinence. Keeping track of your fertile time is important, but timing alone is not a sure enough method. Using fertility awareness along with another method to abstain during the high-risk days is a good idea.

Withdrawal is better than nothing, but it has a high failure rate, disturbs sexual intimacy, and offers no protection against STDs.

Nonmethods

The folklore of birth control is full of weird and worthless ways to prevent, or abort, an unwanted pregnancy. All kinds of potions, notions and motions have been tried. These include sneezing by the woman and breath-holding by the man, driving a car over bumpy roads, and putting various things into the vagina after sex. Since pregnancy only sometimes follows intercourse, almost anything can appear to work for a while, simply on the basis of chance.

Many children are killed each year by running out into the street. But a larger number do it and escape death or injury because no car was coming. That's "dumb luck," not accident prevention! Couples who take no precautions with sex are like kids running into the street. Luck keeps accidents from happening to some, but within a year 85 percent will have a pregnancy (about 10 percent have a fertility problem).

Some people swear by a method that "worked" for them or a friend, but beware! They may be lucky, or they may be sub-fertile — irregular ovulation in the woman, for example, or low sperm count in the man.

DOUCHING

Douching, or washing out the vagina, might seem like a good idea, but sperm move within seconds from vagina to cervix where a douche can't reach. Unfortunately, myths about douching for contraception persist, supported in the past by product mislabeling and phony advertising. Vinegar was often recommended. Women kept it handy for douching after intercourse. As times changed, so did douches: Lots of young women would shake a bottle of cola and squirt it inside.

Douching is not necessary for normal "feminine hygiene." New research leads experts to discourage douching because it can damage delicate vaginal tissue and bring infection into the uterus and oviducts (Zhang et al. 1997). The chemicals in douches can cause genital irritation — sometimes even in males whose girlfriends use them. This is not only annoying, but can increase susceptibility to STDs. The vagina has normal secretions which function to keep it healthy. Soap and water for the perineum (the outside area from vulva to anus) will do the rest. If there is an abnormal odor or discharge, consult a doctor. Unfortunately some women, perhaps prodded by men, think of their vaginas as dirty, and reach for any product which promises to make them "clean." Douches don't.

CONDITIONS OF INTERCOURSE

Timing: Some people believe that there are times when a woman cannot get pregnant if she has unprotected sex. We have already noted that the "safe period" (even during menstruation) is only relatively safe, not guaranteed. Even more risky is the notion that you won't get pregnant the "first time" you have sex. A new mother who breastfeeds her infant may have delayed ovulation but that is not guaranteed, either. Remember:

• A woman has no immunity against pregnancy her "first time." Her risk level depends on where she is in her menstrual cycle at the time of intercourse. Unless she knows there will be no egg present for about five days following intercourse, there is risk, and she cannot know that for sure.

• Unprotected sex during menstruation is safer than at other times, but occasionally an egg is released during the period. No time is totally risk-free. Natural family planning (tracking the cycle carefully and avoiding sex during the fertile interval) tries to reduce that risk, but it has a high failure rate.

• Breastfeeding is a healthful, natural experience for infant and mother, but it cannot be relied upon as a contraceptive. Breastfeeding suppresses ovulation in most women for some time after childbirth, but it is not possible to predict when ovulation will resume. And having another pregnancy when taking care of a new baby is not a good idea. The first menstrual period after childbirth indicates that ovulation has resumed, but that period may never come if you become pregnant again.

Positions: Another myth holds that a woman cannot get pregnant having sex standing up or by keeping one foot on the floor! Untrue. The only position that protects against pregnancy is distance — that is, abstinence.

OTHER MYTHS

Reducing sperm count: Sperm production takes place at a temperature slightly below that of the body — that's why the testicles are in an "outside pocket," the scrotum. (Undescended testicles must be lowered surgically into the scrotum, or the male will grow up to be sterile.) Some people mistakenly believe that taking hot baths or wearing tight undershorts will reduce sperm count: Heat may slow down the process of sperm production, but there will still be millions of sperm waiting to fertilize an available egg.

Lack of orgasm: Some sperm can be released even if a man does not climax inside the vagina. There is a myth that a woman will not become pregnant unless she has a climax. That's false, of course, but as a myth it made sexual enjoyment more difficult for many women who believed it and became afraid to have an orgasm.

Future Methods

While contraceptives today are immeasurably superior to what existed in your parents' and grandparents' generations, there is much room for improvement in birth control and disease prevention. Public and private groups are working to develop new methods. Scientific research takes time, and we don't know how soon new methods will be available. Here are some to watch for.

Barrier Contraceptives

These are of two kinds, mechanical and chemical. Both types help prevent pregnancy and STDs.

Researchers are trying to improve the effectiveness of mechanical barriers while minimizing side effects. *Lea's Shield* is a one-size-fits-all, diaphragm-like device with a one-way valve to allow air to escape during placement. This results in a more secure fit against the cervix. When used with spermicide, it appears to prevent pregnancy at least as well as traditional barriers. However, it is not likely to protect against STD transmission. More research is needed before the FDA decides whether to approve this method. *Femcap* is a silicone rubber device like a cervical cap. It fits comfortably and is not easily dislodged. Available in three sizes, it is fitted by a clinician. Like *Lea's Shield*, it does not protect against STDs. FDA approval should come by the end of the decade. *Diaphragm* improvements are being explored, including a disposable one that releases nonoxynol-9 spermicide. An "easy fit" user-friendly model that can be worn longer is also being studied.

Chemical barriers may not contracept as well as the above, but they may protect better against infection. Much research is being done to find ways to improve existing spermicides (such as nonoxynol-9, the one most commonly used in the United States) and to develop new microbicides that prevent STDs. New microbicides could provide enhanced protection against pregnancy and STDs. Vaginal contraceptive films (VCFs), sponges, and suppositories are under study. *Hormonal methods* are among the better methods we now have: the pill, Norplant, and Depo-Provera. New injectables and implants are under development. *Implanon* is a single implant that lasts for two years. *Norplant II* is an improved version of Norplant that uses only two rods instead of six. Another method under study is the *vaginal ring*, a doughnut-shaped device that releases hormones (progestins) to prevent pregnancy. The user wears it for three weeks and then removes it for a week to allow for menstruation.

Hormones for men are in the works, too. The idea is to temporarily suppress sperm production, but this is still years away from realization. Also, side effects are a problem. For the time being, the only new male contraceptives will be improved condoms.

INTRAUTERINE DEVICES (IUDs)

A *frameless IUD* is in the works. Eliminating the frame removes pressure against the uterus and minimizes cramping. The *Levonorgestrel IUD* is expected to provide seven years of protection. Its main disadvantage will be cost, which is higher than the copper devices. It is already available in Finland, and should gain approval in the United States before long.

VACCINES

"Immunocontraceptives" theoretically would interfere with fertilization by producing antibodies to sperm, for example. This research is in its early stages, and no contraceptive vaccines are expected to be available for some years.

Frequently Asked Questions

Can vasectomies and tubal ligations be reversed?

Sometimes, but not reliably, with microsurgery. The fact that some men and women change their minds after this surgery should be a warning: Don't rush into it. Sterilization is a great method for adults who have either finished having children or have decided they do not wish to have any. It is not recommended for young adults even if they feel strongly that they won't want children later; people do change their minds. You should consider sterilization to be permanent.

Since I started using a diaphragm, my boyfriend doesn't want to use a condom—he says using two contraceptives is overkill. I think the more protection the better. Am I paranoid?

No. You're wise. Using a condom is always a good idea because it is the only method that protects against both pregnancy and sexually transmitted diseases. The diaphragm alone provides good (not excellent) protection against pregnancy; combine it with the condom and you increase protection significantly. Combining methods such as these also allows both partners to play a role in responsible sex rather than letting the burden fall to only one of you.

My friend told me that douches can be used as contraceptives if you add spermicide to the douching solution. Is that true?

No. Sperm enter the cervical canal so quickly after ejaculation that no douching solution can catch all of them. Better to use spermicide as directed—inserted before intercourse begins, along with a diaphragm or condom. If you use spermicide for contraception and insist on douching, make sure you wait six to eight hours after intercourse to avoid washing away the spermicide. Some sperm get into the cervix quickly, but many are swimming around for hours on their way up.

Chapter 12

Emergency Contraception

Postcoital ("after sex") contraception is an emergency because it must be used promptly after unprotected sex. It's not as good as primary contraception, and it's no excuse for taking chances, but it is much better than abortion (which is not contraception, but a remedy for contraceptive failure). Emergency contraception (EC) is secondary prevention. The odd thing is that it mainly prevents worry, since most times that it's used there is no pregnancy — just the possibility of one. But pregnancy is nothing to gamble with, even if the odds are against it. And EC is far easier than abortion.

Jan, 17, and her boyfriend, Ryan, 18, had been going out for nearly two years, and had recently started having sexual intercourse. They always used condoms. But one evening, as Ryan pulled out, he saw that the condom was torn. They were devastated. "Jan and I talked about the risks of having sex, like getting pregnant, but we were really careful and I thought it could not happen to us," explained Ryan. Jan was scared — she had had her period about two weeks before, which meant she might be at her fertile time. She could not sleep all night. "In the morning I called my friend, Ann, who told me there was some kind of 'morning after pill,'" Jan said. But she didn't know how to get it. Jan called a local Planned Parenthood clinic and asked about it. Planned Parenthood told her to come in for an appointment, and they provided her with emergency contraception — high doses of birth control pills. Jan got her period three weeks later — much to her relief and Ryan's.

Jan and Ryan were lucky. They knew right away that their contraceptive had failed and were able to get help immediately to avert what could have been an unplanned pregnancy. Not everyone is so fortunate.

Remember, no contraceptive is 100 percent effective in preventing pregnancy. In fact, 60 percent of all pregnancies that occur in the United States each year are unintended. One half of unintended conceptions result in births, and the other half in abortions.

Researchers estimate that half of these unintended pregnancies occur because of a contraceptive failure — either user error or a faulty method — and half occur because no contraception was used at all. Who is having these unintended pregnancies? Not just teenagers. In 1987, 40 percent of pregnancies among married women were unintended, as were half of those among women aged 20–34, and three-quarters of pregnancies among women over 40. Still, among teens, 82 percent of pregnancies are unintended.

Thoughtful decisions about whether to have sexual intercourse — and correct, consistent use of contraceptives if the decision is "yes" — are essential to prevent accidental pregnancy. Even good contraceptors find themselves vulnerable — a broken condom, an IUD expelled — and the chance of pregnancy suddenly grows from minuscule to very large.

Emergency contraception (EC) is used to prevent pregnancy after unprotected sexual intercourse. It can be requested when you think your method of contraception has failed, if you've been raped, or if no method of contraception was used. *We warn readers that this is not a substitute for regular contraception.* Instead, as its name indicates, it is something for that unfortunate emergency.

The best example of this method is the use of emergency contraceptive pills, or "morning after" pills. Another method is postcoital insertion of an intrauterine device (IUD). These methods provide a safety net or backup for instances where primary prevention fails. We think of them as secondary prevention. But don't be careless about primary birth control: Emergency contraceptives are less effective than primary prevention, and they have some significant side effects. Although we mention both the pill and the IUD, the latter method is generally not recommended for teenagers.

History and Background

Throughout history, women have tried — usually to no avail, sometimes with awful consequences — to prevent conception after intercourse. Some of their practices resulted in infection, infertility and even death. Douching (washing out the vagina) with a variety of substances has been tried for centuries. In ancient Egypt, for example, women douched with wine and garlic. Even today, women have resorted to douching with carbonated and cola drinks. Such efforts are both ineffective and dangerous; these materials are not sterile and can lead to serious pelvic disease.

The first postcoital contraceptive was developed in the 1940s and required a high dose of diethylstilbestrol (DES, a form of estrogen). It was effective in preventing pregnancy; ironically, it proved helpful in preventing miscarriages once pregnancy was established (among women who had difficulty continuing pregnancy). Later, however, DES was found to cause cancer and death, as well as permanent problems for the woman's offspring, and its use was stopped in all circumstances.

Emergency contraceptive pills have been used in Europe for more than a decade, yet few women in the United States know about the method, and even doctors are not well-informed. The main reason is that no company has applied to the U.S. Food and Drug Administration (FDA) for approval to market birth control pills or IUDs as emergency contraceptives. Companies may be concerned that some advocacy or religious groups would say EC was really abortion and protest. Without FDA approval for emergency contraceptive use, manufacturers cannot market pills and IUDs for this purpose — the package labels cannot mention it. However, FDA regulations do allow physicians to prescribe certain regimens of oral contraceptives for emergency contraceptive purposes, and family planning clinics that receive federal Title X (ten) funds can also prescribe them.

According to a survey by the Kaiser Family Foundation, more than two-thirds of obstetricians and gynecologists know about emergency contraceptives and consider them safe and effective. But the majority said they had prescribed the pills fewer than five times in the preceding year. A recent poll of physicians in adolescent medicine reported similar results; over half of these doctors were women. Only 28 percent tell teenage patients about this method during routine health visits.

There is now a hotline number to call for referrals to providers of EC (see "Getting and Using EC," below). In the first nine months it received over 34,000 calls.

Mifepristone (RU 486), the "abortion pill," is not the same as the emergency contraceptive pill. While the former may be taken up to nine weeks into a pregnancy to cause abortion, the latter must be used within three days and prevents pregnancy altogether. (We discuss RU486 in Chapter 13.)

In most instances, unprotected sex does not result in pregnancy, so EC is more often a form of reassurance than a physical remedy. Since it is impossible to tell whether a woman will become pregnant in the first few days after having sex, she can only estimate the risk of becoming pregnant. If sex occurred in the fertile period, that would increase the risk. But ovulation is somewhat unpredictable. Since the emergency pill method is quite simple, it is a good idea to use it in case of doubt. The stress of waiting for your next period is great: If the period is light, you still don't know; if the period is late, it could be due to stress, not pregnancy.

How It Works

Emergency contraceptive pills are high doses of birth control pills that are prescribed by a clinician. These pills are sometimes called "morning after pills," but they can be taken up to three days (72 hours) after unprotected sex. There are several theories about how they work:

• They alter the lining of the uterus to prevent a fertilized egg from implanting in the uterus and growing.

• They inhibit ovulation (release of the egg) in some women.

• They affect the speed at which a fertilized egg passes through the Fallopian tubes.

These effects are temporary and subside soon after you stop taking the single dose of pills.

Emergency contraceptive pills *must* be taken within 72 hours of unprotected sex, that is, before you could be pregnant. Once you are pregnant, they will not work.

Not all birth control pills can be used as emergency contraceptives.

Depending on which type is prescribed, you take either two or four pills immediately, and the same dose again 12 hours later.

Even if you have birth control pills at home, it is important to consult a health care provider before using them as emergency contraceptives. As with any potent medication, there are risk factors and side effects. However, at your appointment you may ask the clinician about extra emergency contraceptives to keep at home in case they are needed in the future.

You should get your period about three weeks after taking the pills. If you do not, see your clinician for an exam and a pregnancy test.

The copper IUD is another emergency contraceptive option. It must be inserted into the uterus five to seven days after unprotected sex. It probably works by preventing a fertilized egg from implanting in the uterus. It may also immobilize sperm or prevent sperm from fertilizing the egg, depending on when in the woman's cycle the sex took place. An added benefit is that the IUD can be left in place for continuing birth control (see Chapter 9).

There are two kinds of IUDs available in the United States: the Copper T 380A and the Progesterone (see Chapter 9). Only the Copper T can be used as an emergency contraceptive. It offers a bigger "window" of opportunity since the IUD is inserted within five to seven days after unprotected intercourse, compared to the three-day limit for the pill.

Effectiveness and Safety

Emergency contraceptive pills prevent approximately 75 percent of pregnancies that would have otherwise occurred, and could therefore reduce the need for abortion by 50 percent.

Many studies have found emergency contraceptive pills to be safe. Even so, they should not be used as routine contraception for several reasons:

• They are not nearly as effective as other methods of birth control.

• They can have significant side effects: About half of women who use them experience nausea and 20 percent vomit. (If you vomit soon after taking the pills, call your health care provider and ask if you should take an additional dose.) Other common side effects are headaches, sore breasts, dizziness, or fluid retention.

As for the postcoital IUD, it appears to be effective as well. In studies of over 1,300 women who have used the postcoital IUD, only one became pregnant.

In general, IUDs are advisable only for women who have had a child: The nulliparous (never-pregnant) woman has a smaller uterus, which will not easily accept the IUD. Infection is not common, but if it does occur it could result in pelvic inflammatory disease (PID), which often leads to infertility. Women with multiple sex partners have a higher risk of infection and should not use the IUD. Of course, women with a history of pelvic infection should also choose a different method.

In rare instances, a woman who cannot use the pill may use the IUD only temporarily for EC, then have it removed and choose another method of ongoing birth control if she is sexually active.

Getting and Using It

The key to emergency contraception is getting it soon enough. These methods are only available with a prescription, so you must get them from a health care provider who can review your medical history and determine if you have any risk factors that would keep you from using either one.

Not all physicians prescribe EC. If yours does, schedule an immediate appointment. If yours does not, or if you have no regular source of health care, or you do not want to reveal your need to your doctor, then a family planning clinic, rape crisis center or hospital emergency room can advise you, if not treat you. But there is also a quick and simple way to find help.

The Emergency Contraceptive Hotline gives information on methods and has the names and phone numbers of about 2,000 providers of EC. When you call, an automated program lists the names and telephone numbers of providers in your area. The hotline number is 1-800-584-9911.

A directory listing health professionals who provide EC has been published on the World Wide Web (see Resources Appendix).

EC and STDs

Unprotected sex puts a woman at risk for disease as well as pregnancy. Emergency contraceptives do not protect against infection. If there is any chance you have been exposed, visit your health care provider and get tested. Left untreated, STDs often have serious consequences.

Conclusion

Emergency contraceptives work to prevent conception and, if conception occurs, to prevent implantation (pregnancy), which explains why you need to use the method as soon as possible after unprotected intercourse — preferably within three days with the pill, and no later than a week with the IUD.

Honor your own beliefs and principles in deciding what to do about a possible unplanned pregnancy. People disagree about when life begins — for some it is at conception (when a sperm fertilizes an egg), for some it is when a fetus is viable (can probably survive outside the womb), and for others it is at birth. And people don't agree about when pregnancy occurs — for some it's at conception, but medically it's considered to be when the embryo implants in the uterus, about three to 14 days after conception. Some people are comfortable with EC because it is used so early on; others feel that disrupting implantation is akin to abortion and avoid it for that reason.

Those who refuse EC on principle will generally refuse abortion if it turns out they are pregnant. In that case they choose to continue the pregnancy and must decide whether to raise the child or make a placement for adoption.

The moral of the story? Avoid risk by *always* using protection. Unprotected sex is a gamble — the risk may be small, but it is never zero. In case of a broken condom or rape, there is help; but while EC is an important backup, it is no substitute for prevention.

Frequently Asked Questions

I wasn't able to use birth control pills as a contraceptive method. Does that mean I can't use birth control pills as EC?

No. Most women in your situation are able to use emergency contraceptive pills safely. However, your clinician will review your medical history and make that decision.

How will I know if EC worked?

Since the odds are that there was no conception, you cannot know whether the method worked. You will know it did not work if signs of pregnancy occur soon. Pregnant or not, your period may not start on time. If it doesn't come in three weeks, see your clinician for an exam and pregnancy test.

What do I do if the pills fail?

Discuss your pregnancy with your doctor, a counselor and/or your parents. You need to decide whether to have an abortion, continue the pregnancy and keep the baby, or make an adoption placement. There have been no long term studies on the impact of emergency contraceptive pills on the fetus. Women who have taken birth control pills without realizing they were pregnant seem not to have a greater risk of a child with birth defects.

Why choose an IUD instead of pills?

Although IUDs are not generally recommended for childless women, there may be some exceptions if:

• It is too late (more than 72 hours after sex) or there is a medical reason to not use the pills;

• You want the most effective emergency method;

• You are opposed to abortion and need to do everything possible to avoid an unplanned pregnancy;

• You want to use an IUD as your ongoing contraceptive.

Contraceptive Methods: An Overview

This chart provides an overview of contraceptive methods. When it exists, STD prevention is mentioned under "advantages." Note the following definitions used in this chart:

Coital: During or immediately before intercourse

Precoital: Hours before intercourse

Postcoital: Shortly after intercourse

Noncoital: Has no time relation to intercourse

Failure rate: Percent of women accidentally pregnant in one year

Perfect use: Method used correctly and consistently

Typical use: As practiced by many couples, includes lapses or errors

Italics are used to show the strong points of the methods.

The data are based on Hatcher, et al. (1994).

Method	How It Works	Failure Rate— Perfect Use	Failure Rate— Typical Use	Advantages	Disadvantages
None	Chance	85%	85%	None	High rate of pregnancy and STDs
Abstinence	No intercourse	*0%*	Unknown	No risk of pregnancy or STDs	Sometimes unrealistic
Male Condom	Barrier	3%	12%	*Male method; latex protects against STDs; combines with other methods*	Coital
Female Condom	Barrier	5%	21%	*STD protection; precoital.*	Somewhat clumsy
Birth Control Pills: combined	Suppress ovulation	*.1%*	5%	*Very effective; noncoital*	Taken daily; prescription only; some side effects

Method	How It Works	Failure Rate— Perfect Use	Failure Rate— Typical Use	Advantages	Disadvantages
Birth Control Pills: progestin-only	Thicken cervical mucus	.5%	5%	For women who cannot tolerate estrogen	Taken daily; prescription only; some side effects
Diaphragm (plus spermicide)	Barrier	6%	18%	*Precoital; some STD protection*	Insertion requires practice
Cervical Cap	Barrier	9% for women who have not given birth	18% for women who have not given birth	Precoital	Not all women can be fitted, e.g. many women who have given birth
IUD	May block conception or prevent fertilization	.1%	2%	Very effective, long term, reversible protection	Increased STD risk; not for women with multiple partners
Norplant	May suppress ovulation; changes cervical mucus	.09%	.09%	*Effective, long-term, reversible protection*	Outpatient surgical procedure; some side effects
Depo-Provera	May suppress ovulation; changes cervical mucus	.3%	.3%	*Effective, long-term, reversible protection*	Shots every 3 months

Method	How It Works	Failure Rate— Perfect Use	Failure Rate— Typical Use	Advantages	Disadvantages
Natural (NFP)	Avoid sex during fertile time of the month	10%	20%	*No side effects; accepted by the Catholic church*	Requires long abstinence and learning about cycle
Emergency Contraception	Blocks conception or implantation	25%	25%	*Postcoital safety net*	Not as effective as other contraceptives; side effects
Spermicides (foam, jelly, film, cream or suppositories)	Kill sperm	6%	21%	Moderately effective alone; enhance other methods; reduce STD risk	Coital, and can be messy
Withdrawal	Reduces sperm entering vagina	4%	19%	Always available; male method	Depends on male's control; interrupts sex
Male Sterilization: vasectomy	Surgery prevents sperm from being released	.10%	*.15%*	Effective, permanent; quick surgical procedure	For those who want no more children
Female Sterilization: tubal ligation	Surgery prevents fertilization	.4%	.4%	Effective, permanent	For those who want no more children

Chapter 13

Pregnancy Options: Parenthood, Adoption, Abortion

Thou shalt not give birth reluctantly.
— Otto Rank

About 60 percent of all pregnancies are unintended in the United States — 82 percent of those to teens. Shocking? Yes. So is the fact that legal abortion is the most common surgical procedure in the United States. The situation is improving: Teen pregnancy, birth, and abortion rates are all dropping. But we have a long way to go.

Pregnant teens face three choices: parenthood, adoption, and abortion. Abortion is the most common choice, adoption the least. Half of teen pregnancies end in abortion (some 400,000 annually). Of those who give birth, less than ten percent make an adoption placement. That leaves about 370,000 who become young mothers, most of them unmarried.

Parenthood

If you are pregnant and decide to carry the pregnancy to term, begin prenatal care immediately. A healthy pregnancy requires some lifestyle changes, such as abstaining from alcohol, tobacco and other drugs that can interfere with the healthy development of the child-to-be.

Becoming a parent is a challenge for even the best-prepared people. In today's world that means mature couples in durable relationships, with a stable loving home, support network, at least one good job, and health insurance. We think it's a bonus if one parent can stay home with the child in the early years. These goals are hard to meet. Many couples try to balance career and parenthood and are constantly pressed for time, money, and energy, although they can still do a good job.

Childbirth begins a new stage in life for parents. And parenthood is largely on-the-job training, and tough training it is. Only a few schools have programs that give a hint of what parenting is like: taking care of a doll that cries at intervals for a day or two, or keeping a raw egg from breaking while you are in charge of it. But parenthood is all this and more.

Parenthood for teens is especially difficult. You must give up your own childhood in order to put the baby first. Many teenagers are raising children with the help of family, friends, boyfriends, community programs, or alone. But most of them say that if they could have another chance, they would postpone childbearing to a time when they are more mature.

Some 70 percent of teen mothers who are still in high school drop out. Many will have more pregnancies, and many will end up on welfare. They and their children will not have good prospects for the future. There are exceptions, of course, and we believe that a good society will provide for all its members. Reducing welfare benefits for poor mothers is punishment, not prevention. There will always be teenagers choosing parenthood even if it is not in their best interest, because they have so little else to look forward to in life. Grownups, including well-educated "solid citizens," make serious mistakes for which they are punished less than teen mothers. Life often isn't fair, but having a child as a protest or as a consolation, while understandable, is still not a good idea. Parenthood is a life-changing event. If the time is right, it's a wonderful change; if the time isn't right, it can be a detrimental one.

Adoption

Pregnant teenagers who are not ready to be parents have two options: abortion or adoption. Abortion may not be an option for some, because of religious or personal values, or because the pregnancy is already too far along. We will take a brief overview of adoption, and then consider abortion.

Many mature couples who are unable to have children are ready and willing to be parents through adoption. There are between one and two million U.S. couples eager to adopt. Since there are only about 30,000 healthy infants placed with adoptive families each year, the demand far exceeds supply, and so many of these childless couples seek infants from other countries. Less than ten percent of births to unmarried women are placed for adoption. Among teens, some estimates are even lower: Between one and five percent of pregnant teens choose to make adoption placements.

While placing your baby may be a difficult decision, women who do so are usually comforted in the knowledge that the child will be raised by adults who are qualified and eager to be parents. State laws require adoptive parents to pass a screening, a home study by a licensed agency or professional. Information is exchanged between birth mothers (and fathers, too) and the adoptive parents; often the birth mother has several couples to choose from. If the birth mother wishes, the adoption process can sometimes be completely open with meetings and continuing contact, at least with letters and photographs.

Adopted children are likely to have social and economic advantages over children who remain with their unmarried birth mothers. A large-scale study of adopted adolescents by the Search Institute in Minneapolis (1994) shows that those adopted early (within the first year) have adjusted very well. Also, birth mothers who postpone parenthood through adoption did well: They had more education, better employment, and were less likely to have another premarital pregnancy than those who kept their babies.

Adoption laws vary from state to state. About two-thirds of all adoptions are arranged by adoption agencies, public or private. A public agency is a state or county agency supported by tax dollars. A private agency is usually licensed by the state but gets its funding from adoptive families and/or charitable donations; many are church-affiliated. Adoption agencies work with pregnant women of all ages who are considering placing their children for adoption and with adults who want to adopt. Some people use an attorney or other intermediary instead of an agency to arrange an "independent adoption." Although most adoption agencies and attorneys meet high standards of professional conduct, including ethics, some do fall short. Be sure to check out the agency you decide to use by contacting your State Adoption Specialist (see the Resources Appendix). Ask whether the professional or agency you plan to contact is licensed and in good standing and whether there are any complaints or investigations on record. Other organizations we have listed in the Resources Appendix can answer a variety of questions about adoption.

Abortion

Induced abortion is a medical procedure done by choice to interrupt an unwanted pregnancy; miscarriage is an abortion that occurs by accident.

There is hardly any subject in the world around us that is as controversial as abortion. For those who believe that a human being exists from the moment of conception, abortion is murder. Those who believe that the fetus is not yet a human being usually support the right of a woman to end an unwanted pregnancy. The laws of most societies, including ours, do not regard a fetus — particularly at the early stages — as a human being. Two cells, egg and sperm, join at conception, and a full-term infant is born nine months (40+ weeks) later. A fetus is usually viable — able to survive birth — after the fifth month (20+ weeks) of gestation, and sometimes earlier. The controversy rages on: Is a fetus an "unborn baby," an "innocent human being," or simply a pregnancy subject to the will of the person upon whom it is dependent?

In an ideal world, abortions would not be needed because all pregnancies would be wanted by the women involved. While many accidental pregnancies turn out well, the health and social risks associated with unwanted or premature pregnancy are a serious problem for individuals, families and society. Our goal in writing this book is to reduce the occurrence of unplanned pregnancy and abortion, but safe medical abortion should be an option when a woman and her physician decide it is in her best interest.

It is a shame that so many abortions are performed every year, but the answer is not prohibition: That has already been tried and it didn't work. Since abortion became legal, U.S. maternal and infant mortality rates have gone down, although these rates are still higher than in other industrialized countries.

History and Background

Until recent times, there was no truly safe method of inducing abortion. Ancient prescriptions and folk remedies did not work reliably and often harmed or even killed the women who used them. Before 1973, legal abortion was available in the United States only when a pregnancy threatened the life or health of the mother. Often the procedure was done for a woman with connections or money, in secret — sometimes safely but often by quacks and charlatans. Many desperate women tried to abort themselves, which is why the coat-hanger has become the symbol of illegal, unsafe abortion. Emergency hospitalization for bleeding and infection — along with sterility and even death — often followed "back alley" abortion.

That changed when, on January 22, 1973, the U.S. Supreme Court ruled in the famous case of *Roe v. Wade* that abortion would be legal throughout the country. Since then, many pieces of legislation have been introduced at the federal, state and local level to try and regulate abortions. These include requirements for waiting periods and parental notification where the patient is a teenager. Such efforts will continue, given the strong feelings on both sides of the abortion issue.

In the near future there is likely to be a significant change in the way women obtain abortions in the United States. The U.S. Food and Drug Administration (FDA) is expected to approve Mifepristone (RU 486) for use in the United States, which could greatly reduce the number of surgical abortions because the same result can be obtained by taking this new medication (explained further, below).

Abortion Trends in the United States

Abortion statistics are not precise because some states have no abortion reporting system. However, the Centers for Disease Control and Prevention (CDC) does compile and collect information provided by states, and their work is supplemented by surveys and research conducted by organizations such as the Alan Guttmacher Institute. Together, these data provide an overview of abortion in the United States.

More than half of pregnancies are unintended, and half of those —
over one-quarter of the total — are aborted. In 1994, 1.4 million abortions were performed, down from about 1.5 million per year in 1992.
Of those, 308,000 were obtained by teenagers. Most women who obtain
abortions are young: 55 percent are under the age of 25, including 22
percent who are teenagers. The highest abortion rate is among 18–19
year olds, who are mostly unmarried and pregnant for the first time.
Abortion-seekers are more likely middle class than poor. All told, 38
percent of women who become pregnant as teenagers choose abortion,
while 62 percent continue their pregnancies to term. Since 82 percent
of teen pregnancies are unintended, it is clear that many girls are having babies they didn't plan for.

Teenagers are a minor part of a major problem. According to *Sex
and America's Teenagers* (Alan Guttmacher Institute, 1994), teens account
for less than one-third of unintended births, nonmarital births, and
abortions each year. Why do women (of all ages) resort to abortion?
For several reasons; the numbers add up to more than 100 percent
because many women have more than one reason:

• having a baby would interfere with work, school or other respon-
sibilities: 75%

• not mature enough: 66%

• cannot afford to have a child: 66%

• do not want to be a single parent or have problems in their relationship with husband or partner: 50%

• fear that the fetus may have been harmed by medications or other
conditions: 12%

• pregnancy resulted from rape or incest: 1 percent (15,000 per year).

What do abortion-seekers say about how they got pregnant? Over
half, 58 percent, report a contraceptive failure. The other 42 percent
used no method of contraception despite their wish not to get pregnant. For this 42 percent, the abortion service often provides the first
counseling in contraception. Although contraceptive use is not fool-
proof, it can reduce the probability of abortion by 85 percent (Henshaw
and Kost).

Access to Abortion for Teenagers

States regulate abortion for teenagers much more than for older women, and much more than for other teen health issues. The U.S. Supreme Court has ruled that a state cannot give parents an absolute veto over their minor daughter's decision to end a pregnancy; states can require parental consent or notification, or permission of a judge, for a minor to get an abortion without her parents' knowledge. Currently, 29 states have laws in effect that require the involvement of at least one parent (or guardian) in the pregnant minor's decision to have an abortion.

At the same time, 45 states and the District of Columbia allow a minor who has delivered a baby to place her child for adoption without her parents' permission or even their knowledge (AGI 1995). A mother, no matter how young, is considered an emancipated minor— one who no longer requires parental involvement in decision-making. But a pregnant girl cannot make a decision to terminate a pregnancy and remain a true minor without a guardian's consent. It's curious and confusing.

Adoption and abortion are both strategies for resolving an unplanned pregnancy. Both are difficult, life-changing decisions, and both involve significant medical procedures (abortion or childbirth). Although these laws seem to encourage adoption over abortion, the success rate is low: One teen mother in ten chooses the adoption route at a time when there is a shortage of babies for adoption.

Even so, the American Academy of Pediatrics takes the position that adolescents have a right to confidentiality:

> **The rights of adolescents to confidential care when considering abortion should be protected. Genuine concern for the best interests of minors argues strongly against mandatory parental consent and notification laws.**

If you think you may be pregnant, find out for sure with a home pregnancy test or with a test at your doctor's office or clinic. Early diagnosis gives you time to consider your options. If you choose to terminate the pregnancy, an early abortion is simpler and less risky. If you choose to continue the pregnancy, starting prenatal care is important for a healthy baby.

The majority of minors (61 percent) have abortions with a parent's knowledge. Younger girls are more likely to tell a parent. Even if you are not required to obtain parental consent, you may still want to, and we encourage it. If you are convinced that the information would only hurt your parents and your relationship with them, or if you are in an abusive family situation, you may want to confide in another adult who knows the family and to whom you can entrust a secret. You can also tell a counselor or social worker. In some cases a "judicial bypass" is possible so that parents are not notified. Getting another perspective in a crisis can be helpful. The decision is yours.

It's scary admitting to your parents that you're pregnant — especially if they'll be shocked to learn you're sexually active — but the sooner it's done, the better. Parents are often more understanding than their children expect; they may even feel guilty for not having provided more guidance along the way. Despite being upset, even angry, parents usually realize that this is no time for reproach and punishment. This is an opportunity for them to demonstrate their understanding and support. If you have done some "homework" and have basic information on abortion services, including cost, your parents will see that you have taken responsible and practical steps toward solving your problem.

> "Telling my parents I was pregnant and thinking about an abortion was the scariest thing I have ever done. They didn't even know I was having sex! I didn't think they'd kick me out of the house or anything, but I was afraid they'd be so mad and upset and I'd end up having to console them when I was the one who needed support and advice. I also thought they'd make me stop seeing my boyfriend, Blake," said 16-year-old Cindy. "Actually, I was really surprised at how cool they were. They said they'd do anything they could to help and that they were really glad I had told them. My mom said it was really important for me to get a more reliable method of birth control to use in the future and we agreed I'd see if I could go on the pill after the abortion. In a way it was a big relief to tell them."

If you feel that your parents will be very upset, you may be able to arrange for the doctor or a counselor to talk with them. Doctors, nurses, and counselors in abortion services have spoken personally with distraught parents more than a few times.

Seventeen-year-old Jessica explained, "My parents and I have just never talked about sex; telling them I was pregnant and getting an abortion was way too much information to be an icebreaker. I didn't tell them, but in some ways I wish I could have."

Finding where to get an abortion is easier in some places than in others. The number of abortion providers has declined in recent years, and 84 percent of all U.S. counties lacked an abortion provider in 1992. Only about half of abortion facilities provide services to women after the twelfth week of pregnancy. If you are having difficulty finding a provider that performs abortions, try contacting a local Planned Parenthood or other health clinic. You also can call the National Abortion Federation.

The cost of a first trimester abortion averages around $300. The U.S. Congress has barred the use of federal funds to pay for abortions for Medicaid-eligible women except when the woman's life would be endangered by a full-term pregnancy or in cases of rape or incest. However, 12 states and the District of Columbia use their own funds to pay for abortions for low-income women.

How Abortions Are Done: Amanda's Story

Chuck and I had been going together for a long time and had always been careful about birth control. I used a cervical cap pretty regularly, but, I admit, not always. Since my periods were irregular, there were times when I thought I might be pregnant. This time I was. A pregnancy test was positive! I had always thought, "If I get pregnant, I'll just get an abortion." But it didn't seem so easy anymore. This was a really big deal. I was terrified—of the procedure, of having regrets, of everything. Thank goodness, there was a clinic not too far away where abortion was part of women's health services. The day after I got my pregnancy test back, I had a counseling session with a nurse there. I decided to go ahead with an abortion. She explained it and I scheduled an appointment for the following week.

Chuck knew about it, but I didn't tell my parents. Chuck and I decided to split the cost. On Thursday I arrived at the clinic for my appointment. Chuck waited in the waiting room; I got changed into a gown and went in another waiting room with about six other women who were getting abortions that morning. About three others looked like students like me and the others looked older. I wondered what each of them was thinking and why they were doing this. There wasn't any conversation. Most were reading or just looking around. I tried doing some homework but it was hard to concentrate.

At 9:30 it was my turn. I was wheeled into the operating room on a stretcher and given an injection to help me relax, since I would be awake during the procedure. My feet were placed in special stirrups at each side of the table and the doctor said I would feel a pinch inside, on my cervix, and then a needle. I did. That was the local anesthetic. Then I just felt a little pulling sensation, and heard the whirring of the vacuum pump. It lasted only a few minutes and then he said that was it. I thanked him, and as they wheeled me out, I looked over to try and see what they had collected in the jar on the vacuum pump. I knew that I was early in my pregnancy, only about eight weeks along, and that there was nothing big enough for me to see. All the same, I needed to see for myself. All I could see in the container was tissue and blood.

I had been in the operating room about 15 minutes. In the recovery room I rested until the nurse came in and checked on me. She told me I could get dressed and that it was time to have a postabortion counseling session. I didn't see why counseling was really necessary. I had already decided to go on the pill. But after meeting with the counselor, I changed my mind. We talked about a lot of things I hadn't expected. She asked me how the procedure had gone and how I felt. Then she asked me about worries or problems associated with the abortion or otherwise. I told her I had been a little afraid of the procedure and of regretting my decision but that I was now so grateful to have had the opportunity to have the abortion. It was the right thing for me.

We talked about contraception and went over my reasons for wanting the pill, how it worked, and how to use it. She also gave me a package of sanitary napkins and said if I was feeling fine — which I was — I could go but that I should take things easy. She gave me a sheet of written instructions about what to do in case of bleeding, pain, fever or discharge. She told me to call her if anything was bothering me, emotional or physical. It was very comforting to feel that they really cared about you. Then Chuck took me home to my house.

I had some cramping that afternoon and bleeding for about two days afterwards, a little heavier than a normal period. The abortion was not a bad experience, but it was not an experience I want to repeat. It's very emotionally and physically draining. I'm glad I'm on the pill now, and I never miss taking it.

Amanda's abortion experience was about as positive as it could be. It was done early, she received excellent counseling, she had a supportive boyfriend, and was empowered to choose a more effective method of contraception to use in the future. While we wish she had told her parents, she had both emotional support and good medical guidance.

Nearly all — 89 percent — of abortions take place in the first trimester (the first three months) of pregnancy, when it is quite safe. Legal abortion is the most commonly performed surgical procedure in the U.S. and is very safe: The risk of death associated with childbirth — also quite low — is ten times that associated with abortion.

At the first appointment you meet with a counselor or doctor to discuss your decision, explain the procedure, and answer any questions. The doctor will also obtain a medical history from you and do a pelvic examination. The abortion will then be scheduled.

The most common method of abortion is vacuum aspiration, which can be performed through the fourteenth week of pregnancy. The patient lies on her back on a table with her knees up, as in a pelvic examination. A local anesthesia is usually given, and sometimes a tranquilizer as well. Using sterile technique to avoid infection, the doctor inserts a very narrow, hollow tube through the cervical opening. This tube is connected to a suction pump, which is turned on as the aspirator tube is moved around inside the uterus, withdrawing its contents within a few minutes. After a few hours of rest the patient is ready to leave. Slight bleeding and cramps may continue for a while.

Another technique, dilation and evacuation (D&E), allows vacuum aspiration to be performed into the second trimester, between the thirteenth and sixteenth weeks of pregnancy. The cervix requires more dilation for this method. For even later pregnancies, a saline injection or other medical method is sometimes used to cause an abortion.

Late abortion (after 26 weeks), although rare, is especially controversial because in the last trimester the fetus is usually viable. Such a procedure is only recommended in extreme cases, e.g., when the fetus is defective and will not live more than a few days, or when there is a serious risk to the mother's health. Sometimes it is done because parents have learned, through genetic testing, that the fetus is abnormal (deformed, for example). Only four in 1,000 (.04 percent) abortions are late. They are, as you can imagine, much more difficult, dangerous, and emotionally traumatic.

The main after-effect of abortion is menstrual-like bleeding that may last one to three days. Almost immediately after an abortion, you may resume normal activities. However, you should refrain from sexual intercourse for several weeks, or until after your next menstrual period. Until the cervix tightens up again, infection of the womb is a slight possibility.

The most promising alternative to surgical abortions is a medical method called RU 486, or mifepristone. When taken with a hormone called prostaglandin, RU 486 causes an abortion. Already being used to abort early pregnancies in European countries and in China, RU 486 is very effective when used within the seventh through ninth weeks of pregnancy.

With the "abortion pill" some people believe we are nearing the end of the era of surgical abortion. Still, the new procedure is not as simple as one might think. The pregnant woman takes one pill to interrupt the implantation (attachment) of the fertilized egg to the uterine wall. Two days later she takes another pill (prostaglandin) which causes contractions and the fetus is expelled, as in a miscarriage. Although a woman could do this in the privacy of her home, and there is very little risk, it can be physically and emotionally uncomfortable. Two weeks later she has a follow-up visit to make sure the abortion was successful, so there are three visits in all. A woman facing the decision about what kind of abortion is better for her has to decide between the physical procedure with anesthetic, which is invasive but quick, or the noninvasive but slower process with the pill.

Conclusion

Any girl who is sexually active needs to think about what she would do if she were to have an unplanned pregnancy. Her options are to have the baby and keep it, make an adoption placement, or have an abortion. This decision is one of the hardest a person ever has to make: Millions of young women face these agonizing choices every year, and most of them become careful users of contraception afterwards. (Let us emphasize that it's much better to never *have* to make that agonizing choice.) Even if you think you know what you would do, in the actual event you may find yourself feeling differently. Abortion, adoption and teenage parenting all have life-changing consequences.

We can't advise you whether or not to have an abortion. Each fully informed woman has the right to make this very personal decision herself. Talk with someone you trust — a counselor, parent, physician, friend, partner (including at least one adult, and one health professional). Just because abortion is an option should not lead to carelessness about contraception. In the crisis of an unwanted or dangerous pregnancy, abortion is a legitimate and safe backup method of birth control, but it is not a substitute for abstinence or contraception. Having unprotected sex because "I can get an abortion" is like riding in a car without wearing a seat belt because "if we have an accident, we can go to an emergency room." Contraceptive failure cannot always be avoided, but having unprotected sex is gambling with your body and your mind.

Frequently Asked Questions

My boyfriend and I disagree about how to handle my being pregnant. He's against abortion and says we should get married and raise the baby together. I can't see doing that at age 16 — I think we're too young. I want an abortion, but he says it's his baby, too, and he should have a say. What do I do now?

It's good to know you can talk frankly with each other about the situation. Each of you deserves to be heard with respect by the other. However, you're the one who is pregnant and would have to carry the baby to term, so you have the final say. The law does not allow a woman's partner to make that decision for her. Have you considered adoption as a compromise? Then you don't take on parenthood at age 16 (your concern) and you avoid abortion (his concern). But he would have to consent to the adoption.

Do Catholic women get abortions?

Yes, in substantial numbers, although their church forbids it. A survey of abortion patients found that about 37 percent of the group were Protestant and 31 percent were Catholic. Four out of five Catholics think that abortion can be a morally acceptable choice in some circumstances. More than half believe that the practice should be legal in many or all circumstances. These attitudes are quite similar to those of people of other faiths. Religion and abortion are both deeply personal issues, so each woman has to decide for herself whether she can reconcile the two. The organization Catholics for a Free Choice provides information and support for those in the faith who accept abortion as legitimate and moral. (See Resources Appendix.)

Will having an abortion affect my ability to become pregnant in the future? Does it increase the chances of breast cancer?

No. Women who have first-trimester vacuum abortions have no greater risk of fertility problems than other women. Abortions performed in the second trimester pose a slightly greater risk, but even then severe complications are extremely rare. Some two dozen studies have examined the link between abortion and breast cancer, with no clear consensus.

Is it true that women who have abortions often regret it and even have psychological problems afterwards?

Although a period of grieving is normal, regrets are rare. There is talk of "postabortion trauma" and long-term consequences, but this is promoted by abortion opponents, unsupported by scientific evidence — and never compared with the consequences of unintended parenthood. Studies have found no significant postabortion effects: A recent study of 5,000 U.S. women followed for eight years found no evidence of widespread postabortion trauma. Abortion is psychologically painful and difficult, but the untoward physical and emotional consequences of premature parenthood are much more common and more serious.

Chapter 14

Mind and Body

*Our bodies are our gardens, to the which
our wills are gardeners.*
—Wm. Shakespeare, *Othello*

Sex is a biological drive shaped by learning, especially in humans. All creatures learn, but humans, thanks to language, have evolved to the point where attitudes and values are stronger than instincts. To us, but not to other animals, sex can be beautiful or ugly, true or false.

In this chapter we consider body and mind (intellect, emotion, and soul) in relation to sex. Sex is complicated on many levels at any age. We have selected some key issues concerning, but not limited to, young adults: the meaning of sex, homosexuality, masturbation, pornography, mental health and illness (including suicide), disorders of sexual function, sexual offenses, body image, social pressures, hygiene and grooming.

What Is Sex For?

Sex serves two major purposes, love (conjugal) and reproduction (procreative). The first concerns relationship (the pleasure bond between two people), while the latter concerns having babies and maintaining the species. Managing these two aspects of sex is a major issue for individuals and societies, philosophies and religions.

These two values of sex can be separated, and usually are. Pregnancy is not the goal of sex for most people most of the time. In order to enjoy sex for its relational value without the consequence of pregnancy, people use contraception or natural family planning.

Sex is a meeting of body and soul. It is said that the body is the house or temple of the soul. This simple but profound metaphor applies to sex. We owe it to our souls to take care of our bodies, and we owe it to the souls of our partners to respect their bodies.

In sexual intimacy we share parts of ourselves that are ordinarily hidden, private. These parts are associated with great sensitivity: in childhood, with embarrassment; in adolescence, with excitement, but also with mixed feelings of desire and anxiety. We are also sensitive about inviting someone into our homes or rooms. Finding a partner with whom you are comfortable anywhere, public or private, in good times and bad, is one of life's great joys. It cannot be rushed, because it requires judgment.

Sex is a strong force in and among most of us. Despite what you often see on TV, most people control their sexual impulses quite well. That doesn't mean they all have happy sex lives. As with driving a car, most people do it safely but it doesn't take much loss of control to cause an accident. Our society has far too many accidents, both traffic and sexual.

Sometimes control is too weak, sometimes too strong, but usually it's about right. Almost everyone feels upset, uncertain, or troubled about sex from time to time. Understanding grows slowly, with experience and maturing judgment. A paradox of modern times is that kids are biologically ready for sex long before they are psychologically ready.

Grownups have a hard time talking to kids about sex for several reasons. First, it's very personal. Second, the awakening of sexual feelings coincides with greater need for independence as adolescence leads toward adulthood. Third, teens are in an unstable, often unpredictable place in life; sometimes you want adult advice and sometimes you want to figure things out on your own.

Most teens want to be treated like adults while they are learning to be adults. Your parents and teachers, clergy and counselors, and doctors were once teens, but they—we—have matured and see the world quite differently now.

Teen Mental Health

What is a mentally healthy teenager? One who has good relationships with family and friends, who gets schoolwork and chores done, who enjoys life and likes her- or himself most of the time, who avoids unnecessary trouble, and who takes responsibility.

Adolescence (Latin: "growing up") is the period from puberty to physical maturity. Some people say that this stage of life is typically American: something emphasized, exaggerated, maybe even invented in the United States. Think of all the products made for or aimed at you: clothes, hair and body care, food and drink, music, TV, cars, cigarettes.

Your language, mood swings, likes and dislikes, fads and fashions — all make our heads spin. You want to be like others yet unique, to be accepted and independent at the same time. That makes your heads spin, too.

Puberty starts earlier and social maturity comes later. Adolescence really lasts from 10 to 25. To succeed in the family and workplace of the 21st century you need more preparation and rehearsal than your parents and grandparents did. Some evidence: The average age at marriage has jumped several years in a generation, and often you can't even rent a car if you're under 25.

The teen years are full of turmoil. Sexual themes and pressures are "out there" more than ever. Best friends come and go. Promises are made, some are kept, others broken. Excitement and boredom, success and failure, joy and heartbreak, independence and attachment, defiance and conformity all somehow go along together. Kids feel life surging all around with tremendous power and they learn it is fragile, too: Accidents take their toll. Serious sexual learning begins.

In folklore and in psychology, sex and mental illness have often been linked — and often wrongly. Deviation from norms has been prohibited in most cultures at various times. All societies try to regulate sexual behavior and reproduction. Abnormality is regarded as illness or crime, and it is treated or punished, whether it is homosexuality, promiscuity, exhibitionism, etc. Attitudes and rules change, and progress is made. For example, there is a greater acceptance of homosexuality, but many people were — and still are — persecuted because they are different, even though no harm to others can be shown to come from this.

Homosexuality was once, but is no longer, considered a mental disorder. In 1973 the American Psychiatric Association removed it from its list of diagnoses. A few professionals will still argue that it's an illness, and some religions declare it a sin. For centuries homosexuals have been persecuted. They tried to hide, often by marrying and raising families while never finding sexual fulfillment. Experts today believe sexual orientation is inborn, a biological (genetic) trait, not under the control of will, although influenced by circumstances. The expression of this trait depends in part on how one is raised, and the environment.

Some people worry about homosexuals being in professions like teaching, medicine, the military and the ministry. Since the trait is apparently inborn, there is little likelihood of anyone being persuaded to change from hetero- to homosexual. Harassment by homosexuals is probably less common than by heterosexuals in similar positions; it is homosexuals who have been subject to unfair discrimination.

Women often suffer discrimination in male-dominated society. Many men have mixed feelings about women's sexuality, dividing them into categories of sexy vs. maternal, or whore vs. Madonna. Men are insecure about paternity, too. When a child is born, we know who the mother is, but there may be doubt about which man is the father. As a result, men have been anxious to control their women. Sexual freedom for men is tolerated more than for women: This is called the double standard. Even today, women who have pregnancies out of wedlock are criticized much more than the men who are equally responsible for those pregnancies.

Sexual Solitaire

Well into the 20th century, medical experts as well as church authorities condemned masturbation — solitary sex, or self-pleasuring — as dangerous and evil. "Self-abuse" and "self-pollution" were the terms applied, along with "solitary vice" and "onanism." In the Bible story (Genesis 38:9), Onan refused to impregnate his brother's widow, instead spilling his seed upon the ground. Onan was slain by God for refusing to father a child, not for masturbation.

In 1995 the Surgeon General of the United States, Dr. Joycelyn Elders, had to resign after saying that masturbation could be part of a sex education curriculum. That message is not yet politically acceptable, even when we know that self-pleasuring is normal for most people, teens and adults. Medical experts today regard masturbation as a harmless, probably helpful, part of healthy human development.

However, it also requires some care. An embarrassing reason to have to go to the doctor is to have an object removed from the genital area, or an injury or infection treated that resulted from masturbation. Genital tissues are delicate, sensitive and — don't forget — relatively clean (compared with unwashed hands, for instance). One erotic practice is especially dangerous: causing a temporary blackout by tightening a rope around one's own neck during masturbation. Called sexual asphyxia, this practice is believed to cause hundreds of deaths each year.

Done sensibly, self-pleasuring won't harm you. It may make you guilty even if your religion doesn't call it sin, perhaps because it feels like a failure of will or of self-control. But if masturbation takes the place of casual sex with others, or going to prostitutes, or even having premature sex with someone you love, then it would seem to be a responsible *and* healthy choice, even a form of self-control. By prohibiting masturbation, or scaring people away from it, authorities only increase the likelihood that sexual intercourse — premature, selfish and risky — will take place.

Normal masturbation is a form of rehearsal. Fantasy is part of it. If you study a musical instrument or a team sport, you will practice your skills alone as well as play with others. The same can be said of sex — finding out how your body responds, and what goes on in your mind as it does. Some may object that it's unnatural because it doesn't make babies. Well, it is natural in that other members of the animal kingdom do it. And it may be particularly important for humans because, unlike other species, our sexual urges are not regulated by estrous (female readiness for pregnancy). We are sexually ready most of the time after puberty, and many people will feel better and be more socially responsible if they have a choice other than sex with a partner or total abstinence.

What about pornography? Its chief purpose is arousal, without any real emotional connection. It may be harmless to the curious, but it can become compulsive (sexual arousal won't occur without it). It tends to simplify and dehumanize sex. Most pornography treats women as objects to please men. Norman Mailer, no prude, wrote:

A sixteen-year-old boy closeted in the bathroom with the photo of a prostitute is laying the physical ground of his neurosis—he will pay later in bad reflex, pinched orgasm and nervous guilt, but at least he is not looking for a fetish—on the contrary, he is beginning the search for a mate. ...

Pornography gives no preparation for sex. In the pornographic dream, all comings come together, the torso is lithe, the smell is clean, pleasure arrives like manna. What a shock for the sensitive adolescent when he finds the courage to capture his first sex... there are dead small corners for which he is not prepared, and responsibility he never knew. Nothing in the life of his fantasy prepared him for tenderness...

—*Advertisements for Myself* (1959)

Many men (and some women) keep this fantasy alive into adulthood. Would there be strip joints, hard-core films, and prostitution otherwise? These are unhealthy ways to be sexual.

Mental Illness and Suicide

This large topic is sometimes, not always, related to sexual issues, so we discuss it briefly. Adolescence is a period of such rapid change that a diagnosis of mental illness is sometimes difficult. It takes more than one sudden mood change or an episode of abnormal behavior like shoplifting, explosive anger, or running away. These are serious enough, though, to warrant evaluation if repeated.

Schizophrenia and other forms of psychosis may make their first appearance in late adolescence, sometimes without warning. The signs include delusions, hallucinations, paranoia, total withdrawal, or inappropriate speech and behavior that show a loss of contact with reality or an abrupt change in personality. Intoxication with alcohol and other drugs can result in psychosis.

According to recent studies, about half of teenagers have thought of suicide at some time, female (62 percent) more than male (44 percent). Five to ten percent reported making suicide attempts, but only three percent sought professional help as a result.

Suicide is the third leading cause of death among teenagers and young adults. As you can see, however, it is not unusual for suicidal thoughts to occur; in fact, they may not be abnormal or dangerous in itself. Such thoughts are a sign of distress, depression, and anxiety, but these feelings come and go. Many creative and successful people have had suicidal thoughts, including Mark Twain, the philosopher William James, and psychiatrist Karen Horney. Those who commit, or even attempt, suicide are a small proportion of those who sometimes think about it.

If someone thinks about it a lot, or has suffered a major setback in life — death of a loved one, breakup of a relationship, having an unwanted pregnancy, being taunted about homosexuality — the risk of suicide goes up. Other factors which increase the likelihood of suicide are illicit drug use and delinquent behavior. People who talk about suicide should be taken seriously. (There is a myth that talking about it means a person won't do it.)

Other signs of distress for which referral to a mental health professional is a good idea: major change in mood, deterioration in school performance, withdrawal from friends and activities, major forms of risk-taking, outbursts of uncontrolled emotion, running away from home, lying, obsessions (such as eating disorders — see "Body Images," below) and complaints of physical symptoms for which no physical cause can be found.

Psychiatrists are physicians who specialize for at least three additional years in the study of emotional disorders. In addition to prescribing medicines and admitting patients to hospitals, they may also work in offices and do psychotherapy, behavior modification, and hypnosis. Clinical psychologists and social workers do not go to medical school but have extensive training in psychological diagnosis and treatment.

Psychotherapy, or the "talking cure," is practiced by these and other mental health professions (psychiatric nursing, marital therapy, counseling). Be careful when you choose a professional in this field. A professional degree and state license should help you decide whether a person has adequate training: Look for a Ph.D. in psychology, MSW in social work, and RN in nursing, for example. If in doubt about a professional's credentials, contact your nearest mental health association, university psychology clinic or medical school psychiatry department. Hotlines are a good bet for referral information.

Sexual Problems

Proof of the power of mind over matter comes from the fact that, as powerful as the sex drive is, it often fails, or is disrupted in some way, despite the wishes of the people involved. Sometimes this is a sign that people aren't ready, but it happens to people at all stages of life. Sexual problems include lack of interest, impotence, frigidity, and premature ejaculation.

Lack of interest may or may not be a problem. Insecure people have the most to say about their sexual conquests, so don't compare yourself with others, especially those who brag. In general, sexual feelings in everyday life are a barometer of general feelings. If you are depressed, angry at your partner, grieving for a lost love, sick, or passionate about something else, you may not have energy left for sexual feelings. If you are afraid of letting someone else be close to you, have guilt about sex, or are attracted only to the "wrong" people, then counseling with a professional may be in order.

Impotence refers to the male's inability to get and maintain an erection. It happens to every male at times. It can be upsetting but also gives a clue to feelings that complicate the sexual picture. If he is too worried about the symptom and sets out to prove himself, "performance anxiety" may make things worse. A casual pickup does not provide a good test of potency, nor does a pornographic film of nonrelational sex; a better one is a relaxed fantasy of loving sex with an appropriate partner. Impotence can have psychological or physical causes.

Lack of arousal, and particularly of orgasm, in the female used to be called frigidity. Sexual readiness usually comes later for her than for him. This is partly a matter of biology, partly social context. Female arousal depends more on the relationship and on delicate shades of emotion. Even the experience of orgasm varies from one time to the next or from one person to the next. Some girls have arousal and release but no dramatic climax. Some women have multiple orgasms (most men have a period of sexual exhaustion after orgasm). If a woman has a considerate partner, she can guide him to increase her enjoyment, and, of course, any woman who wants to can practice by herself.

Premature ejaculation is a common problem with younger men who are easily excited and who do not have much control over their arousal. It can be frustrating for both partners, because the climax may occur within seconds of starting intercourse. It may be a sign of insecurity or discomfort. The treatment involves slowing down the whole sexual process, which can be practiced alone or with a partner.

Other sexual problems include the compulsive need to have props of various kinds (including pornography and drugs) or to talk about fantasies in order to be aroused. Variety is fine, and whatever both partners want is generally all right, but if one partner does not want to do something, it's not right to force it. Strong persuasion borders on harassment and is not part of healthy lovemaking.

Crimes

We have addressed a number of relationship problems in Chapter One. Some of them — violence, cruelty, infidelity — are very serious. Staying in a "sick" relationship means living with abuse. If you cannot leave such a relationship, you should get professional help. Abuse leading to injury and even death usually has been building up for years. Most rape, molestation, and murder is committed by relatives or acquaintances.

Sexual harassment, obscene teasing, and unwelcome touching are all signs of disturbance and should be dealt with strictly. Unwanted touching is called "battery" under the law, and rape, including "date rape," is an extreme form of such behavior. A woman is not responsible for a man's criminal behavior. On the other hand, women should remember that some men blame the woman for their own sexual feelings, and some will take advantage of any sexual opportunity. Use due caution in sexual situations.

Prostitution among teenage girls is a tragic problem. "Imagine you're a young girl in Smalltown, U.S.A," says psychologist and lawyer Marsha B. Liss. "Some guy picks you up in the mall and says, 'Hey, baby! Want to go to Vegas with me?' He befriends you, takes you out for some nice dinners and eventually gets you to Las Vegas. Once you get there, you discover how you're really going to pay for the hotel room: prostitution." A pimp is the man who recruits and manages the prostitute. If you know of such activities, contact the U.S. Department of Justice, Child Exploitation and Obscenity Section.

While we believe in respecting the privacy of consenting adults, we disapprove of sexual or other behaviors that involve force or violence, cruelty, coercion, and invasion of privacy. Rape, molestation, voyeurism (peeping), harassment, stalking and exploitation — taking advantage of the very young, or the intellectually or emotionally handicapped — are, or should be, treated as crimes.

Females tend to develop strong sexual feelings later than males, though in other ways they may mature faster. This creates problems of balance. One-third of girls who had sex at 15 or younger report that the male was 18 or older. They are not well-matched — a three year age difference in the teen years is much more significant than later on. Statutory rape laws are designed to prevent exploitation of younger girls and boys by adults (over 18).

Body Image

The obsession with physical appearance in our society seems to push some people over the brink: Over ten percent of college-age women go through a serious eating disorder. *Anorexia nervosa* is self-starvation, leading to death in 15 percent of cases. *Bulimia* is an illness in which the person binges and then purges by vomiting or use of laxatives. The causes are not well understood.

In anorexia, rare in males, the patient believes that even the smallest items of food will cause unacceptable weight gain. They get no pleasure from eating, only anxiety; their families are worried and upset. Bulimics get some pleasure, or at least some relief of anxiety, by indulging, but then punish themselves by purging. In extreme anorexia a girl gets no comfort by looking at her scrawny body, although she may agree that other girls, although heavier, are thin enough. This is a clear indication of a distorted body image, and calls for psychiatric help.

Diet and exercise shape our bodies as much as anything, given the basic structure determined by our genes. A few points bear emphasis:

• Weight gain results from an intake of calories that is greater than the expenditure; the reverse results in weight loss.

• Fat should provide less than 30 percent of calories, but a low-fat diet can still add weight if you take in too many total calories. Excess carbohydrate calories, e.g., those from sugar and starch, will be converted to fat in the body.

• Crash dieting has a high failure rate. Starvation causes stored fat to be broken down into sugar, and the process can make you sick if it goes too rapidly. Getting to a stable weight takes time.

• Regular, even moderate, exercise helps control appetite. Muscle tissue has a high metabolic rate, which is why people who exercise can eat more without gaining weight.

Women do not begin menstruation (or continue it) if body fat falls below 17 percent: Severe anorectics do not have their periods (*amenorrhea* is the medical term; problems in bone development may result due to lack of estrogen). Another area of concern to most women at some time in their development is breast size; breast tissue is mostly fat. Fashions change concerning body shape. You only have to look at how highly-paid models look from one decade to the next. Unfortunately, many women are displeased with what nature provided, and there are industries and advertisers making a great deal of money from these insecure women. Consider the sad story of silicone breast implants, used by millions of women, many of whom suffered painful and dangerous side effects. A survey conducted by *Self* magazine (May 1996) found that 63 percent of large-breasted women feel self-conscious, and 35 percent of small-breasted women feel less confident. A majority of the 4,000 women who responded would change their breasts if they could, and 58 percent have been taunted or teased because of their breasts.

Boys, too, worry about their bodies, though not as much. They are concerned about muscle bulk and shape and, of course, penis size.

> **The "average" penis is about six inches overall when erect and about 3½ inches round, but penises come in all sizes— larger ones are spectacular but no more effective except as visual stimuli. Smaller ones work equally well in most positions ... men should learn not to give it a second thought.**
> —Alex Comfort, *The Joy of Sex* (1972)

The most sensitive part of the penis, near the tip, goes into the relatively insensitive upper vagina during intercourse, while the clitoris, the most sensitive female part, is just outside the vagina. Men often think that deep penetration excites women, but pubic area contact is more likely to be pleasurable. A larger penis gives no advantage in lovemaking and may be a disadvantage when a woman is physically small and has never borne a child.

Both men and women can be victimized by quack "remedies" to enlarge the penis or the breasts. Creams, salves and herbs don't work, and they are not needed. If you have real concern about an abnormality, males should consult a urologist, females a gynecologist.

Body image themes dominate TV and movie dramas and advertising. What does it take for a guy to get a beautiful girl, and for a girl to get a handsome guy? What about most of us, the average-looking? How do we compete? Are we doomed to lose in the happiness sweepstakes?

No! If good looks and sex appeal were so important in the long run, movie stars and models would never get divorced. So keep your perspective: The beauty that makes good relationships great and long-lasting is deep inside, missed by the casual observer.

Hygiene

Not all germs are bad. Normally, our skin, mouths, and intestines have many bacteria; the vagina has some, and keeps itself relatively clean with secretions. Keeping clean—bathing, brushing teeth, washing hands—is important, but we can't disinfect the parts of our bodies that aren't already germ-free. When you have blood drawn from a vein the technician cleans the spot first with alcohol, which is as close as we can get to disinfecting skin. That disinfection lasts a minute or two. Soap and water don't sterilize the skin, nor do mouthwash or douching eliminate germs, even though they kill or wash away "millions." There will be millions more, mostly harmless, in a few minutes.

The germs we worry about are the ones that often cause infections; they are called pathogens. Cleanliness keeps the number of microbes, including pathogens, at a reasonable level so the body's defenses don't get overwhelmed. Washing keeps germs from accumulating around weak spots or breaks in the skin, just as dental flossing and brushing keeps them from building up in plaque.

Young people are more concerned with bad breath than with cavities—otherwise they would not eat breath sweeteners and chew gum containing sugar. Bacteria love sugar, so in the long run plain water, regular brushing, and flossing are best for keeping your teeth healthy. The amount of toothpaste is not important; the length of time you brush is. The mouth is one of the "dirtiest" parts of the body in terms of germ count. Smoking makes it taste and look dirty.

Another haven for germs is the skin, particularly the scalp and other hairy places. But shampooing can be overdone: *Consumer Reports* finds that a second application of shampoo is wasted since the first one gets the dirt out. Our national obsession with being clean and odorless also leads to overuse of deodorants, mouthwash, and douches. The mouth can never be free of germs and the vagina takes care of itself, so most people can do well with less of these products.

The makers of mouthwash don't tell you this, but some major causes of bad breath come from our lungs, not our mouths, and no amount of mouthwash will prevent it. Onion, garlic and alcohol are the best examples. For a couple of hours after you ingest these things, you will exhale their byproducts from your lungs. Breath fresheners won't help because breathing pumps the "fragrance" out of your lungs. After a few hours the odors are gone. Some may be left in your mouth — after sleep, for example — because the chemicals dissolve in saliva, and then brushing your teeth will help. Smoking also makes your breath foul.

The body secretions — saliva, sweat, skin oils, mucus, seminal fluid, even urine — are normally sterile when they are made and released. Once released, they mix with germs from the body or the air and they will no longer be sterile; in a few hours their odors will change due to bacterial growth. Bacteria and fungi love warm, dark, moist places. The underarm (axilla), crotch, feet, and buttocks-crease are favorite places for germs. Daily washing with soap and water should prevent problems for most people.

Knowing something about germs and using common sense will help you avoid infection. The common E. Coli, a necessary part of the work of the gut, is abundant in fecal material and becomes harmful only if it strays into the urethra, bladder, vagina, etc. Wiping from front to back after going to the toilet is appropriate. Also, the mouth is a germy place, and bite wounds can be nasty because germs enter breaks in the skin. It doesn't take a bite, either: A small nick from a tooth, or a prior cut or broken blister, can be a welcome mat for germs.

Shaking hands, holding hands, and kissing all spread germs, usually without causing infection. The germs are so common that we all have most of them already. You are at risk only if someone has a pathogen (such as flu, herpes, or mononucleosis), or you have a break in your skin where contact is made (hand, face, gum). Sex spreads germs, but not dangerously between partners who are free of STDs, faithful to each other and who keep reasonably clean. Be careful to clean thoroughly if you practice anal sex.

Risk-Taking Psychology

Teenagers often flaunt their indifference to risk. They seem not to worry about the risk of cancer from smoking or sunburn, or being hurt by drinking and driving, or not wearing a seat belt, or by having unprotected sex. Because it's not "cool" to be anxious, many kids shrug and let the grownups worry. (To use psychological terms, adolescents displace their anxiety onto adults.) Most of the time the bad consequence is not felt — at least not right away: Cancer takes a long time to develop; wearing a seat belt is a kind of insurance against an unlikely event; and most unprotected sex does not result in pregnancy. By taking chances and "getting away with it," teenagers boost their sense of security or invulnerability. But on a statistical basis these behaviors have bad consequences, most of them preventable.

Accidents take a large toll in lives and disability among teenagers. Alcohol is a major contributor. Auto accidents are far and away the leading cause of death in the 15 to 24 age group, and males have 80 percent of the casualties. There is a gray area between accident and suicide; sometimes a major depression or anxiety about a relationship contributes to reckless driving. Anyone who fails to use a seat belt or who drinks and drives is playing statistical roulette: The chances of death or injury go way up. We see an exact parallel between seat belt use and safe sex: People who ignore precautions act as though they are invulnerable, yet suffer the most consequences.

Sanity in a Mad World

A free society presents hazards as well as opportunities. This is especially true in the arena of sex. There is nothing more personal or private than sex, yet we see around us many examples of impersonal sex. Movies and television show sexual images and examples to a mass audi-

ence. That's one kind of impersonal sex. Another is instant intimacy —
sex at first sight.

Generally, what two consenting adults do in private is their business, if it does not infringe on anyone else's rights. The sexual content
of TV and movies is often inappropriate for children and offensive to
many adults, but finding ways to regulate it has not been easy.

Freedom goes hand in hand with responsibility: More of one
requires more of the other. Sex has profound physical and emotional
consequences, joyful as well as painful. Adolescence is a time of change,
self-doubt, self-definition, and more. Sex is one piece of the puzzle, and
figuring out where it fits and when you're ready for it can be difficult.
You must know enough and be secure enough to govern your instincts
wisely. Sex is a great source of energy, life and love. You will continue
to learn about it throughout life.

> Sex contains all, bodies, souls,
> Meanings, proofs, purities, delicacies....
>
> Without shame the man I like knows and avows
>   the deliciousness of his sex,
> Without shame the woman I like knows and avows hers.
> —Walt Whitman, "A Woman Waits for Me"

Chapter 15

Discussion and Curriculum Guide

This book is addressed to readers of mid–high school level, omitting material that appears in biology and health courses (e.g., anatomy and physiology of reproduction, glossary of formal and colloquial terms), while emphasizing what is often bypassed. This chapter contains some thought-provoking questions (offered immediately after each subhead) and interesting ideas from several academic disciplines for teachers, advanced students, parents, and librarians. The possibilities are many — our examples only suggestive — to show how "sex contains all," and vice versa.

The discovery of our own sexuality changes us forever. From that moment on we spend much time, thought, and energy enjoying, suffering and controlling its mysterious power. Of course sexual learning is physical and emotional, grounded in experience and relationships, but intelligent reflection and discussion have their essential place. The leadership of good teachers and writers is a great help at a time when the mass media treat sex mostly as seduction and scandal in a context of unreality.

A story is told about the man who read so much about the dangers of smoking that he finally decided to give up reading. Smoking is a harmful addiction that has little in common with sex, except that many teens experiment with both at about the same time. Our purpose here is to take the reading-smoking joke and turn it around. We want the energy of sexual interest to draw the adolescent toward learning. We want to present ideas about sex that are so valuable that students will become addicted to reading and learning in general.

In the last 250 years modern society has evolved from one based in agriculture to an industrial one, and now to the information society in which we find ourselves. The technical material in this book is more than parents can be expected to know — even more than most teachers, librarians and physicians will master. Young people don't need to know it all, but they need to know how to find out what is important and useful.

History

- Has adolescence always been a time of sexual turmoil? How have people — societies, religious and medical authorities, artists — dealt with sexual awakening throughout history?
- Do STDs carry a worse stigma than other diseases? If so, why?
- Is anorexia a modern form of hysteria?

A rich source of information is *Medical History of Contraception* by Norman E. Himes (Gamut, 1963, introduction by Alan Guttmacher). There are many histories of sexuality, feminism, homosexuality, and now one of adolescence: Marcel Danesi's *Cool: The Signs and Meanings of Adolescence* (Univ. of Toronto Press, 1994), which takes a semiotic approach to the development of teenagerhood over the last half-century.

Studies in the history of medicine and psychology are valuable. One of the most dramatic psychiatric illnesses, hysteria, is the subject of several excellent books. The hysteric, usually a woman, is excitable, irrational, and may have physical symptoms like weakness, fainting, paralysis, or blindness. From ancient times hysteria was considered a female disorder caused by wandering of the uterus (*hysteros* in Greek) inside her body. Freud viewed hysteria as the product of repressed memories or wishes about sex. There is renewed interest in the subject as a factor in psychosomatic illness, and in hypnotic susceptibility (recovered memory and the problem of false memory). Elaine Showalter's *Hystories: Hysterical Epidemics and Modern Culture* (1997) is a recent example. Another, more general reference is *Sexual Knowledge, Sexual Science: The History of Attitudes to Sexuality*, edited by Roy Porter and M. Teich (Cambridge, 1994).

Sir William Osler said that if you know syphilis, you know medicine. Thanks to penicillin, most doctors rarely see this disease any more; its deadly mantle may have been passed along to AIDS. Spread chiefly through sex but also through the placenta from an infected pregnant woman to her fetus, syphilis attacks various parts of the body — blood vessels, heart, spinal cord and brain — over a course of years. In the 1800s, most incurable patients in mental hospitals ("insane asylums," in those days) were victims of advanced syphilis, which often produced the aberrations of grandiosity portrayed in Napoleonic caricatures. Until scientists discovered its cause (*Treponema pallidum*, in 1905), many people attributed the symptoms of syphilis to degenerate living or bad genes: drunkenness, drugs, filth, diet, sex. (See, for example, *Ghosts*, by playwright Henrik Ibsen.) There are many excellent histories of medicine, and several periodicals such as *The Bulletin of the History of Medicine*.

Art

- What is pornography?
- How and where should the line be drawn between the interests of artistic expression and those of maintaining standards of decency in the community?

The human body has long been a subject for artists, though some cultures forbid any graphic images. *Ars Medica*, from the Philadelphia Museum of Art (1985), is a catalog of a wonderful exhibit on human health and illness through the ages. Art galleries have had a tacit role in sex education for centuries. Reporting on a visit to the Uffizi Gallery in Florence, Mark Twain wrote: "There are pictures of nude women which suggest no impure thought — I am well aware of that. I am not railing at such. What I am trying to emphasize is the fact that Titian's Venus is very far from being one of that sort. Without any question it was painted for a bagnio and it was probably refused because it was a trifle too strong" (*A Tramp Abroad*).

Religion and Ethics

- If the great religions don't always agree about what is right and wrong, how are ordinary people supposed to know?
- What makes people ethical — love, fear, religion...?

Freedom of religion and separation of state and church are fundamental principles of our society. Thomas Jefferson was a powerful spokesman for these ideas: "Say nothing of my religion. It is known to God and myself alone. Its evidence before the world is to be sought in my life: if it has been honest and dutiful to society the religion which has regulated it cannot be a bad one" (*Works*, VII).

We respect and defend the right of each person to maintain a position as long as others have the same right. We object to coercion, to the imposition of religious doctrine in a democratic society that guarantees freedom of religion. When does the soul come into existence? This is a religious and philosophical problem that we discuss here from the standpoint of tolerance. We take the issue of abortion because it is one of the most difficult and divisive in our country today.

Prior to 1973, abortions could be performed legally in some states, but in others only to save the life or health of a pregnant woman. More often they were performed illegally by amateurs and quacks. Reputable doctors had little training or experience performing abortions. Desperate women who could not afford a baby risked their lives to obtain abortions. Half the sickbeds in gynecology wards of public hospitals were occupied by women with postabortion trauma or infection: Some died, while many required hysterectomies and lost the chance to become pregnant again. In our society, and in many if not most religions, abortion is neither murder nor mortal sin. Murder is a felony but abortion is legal. A fetus is neither a baby biologically nor a person under the law. Terms like "unborn baby" and "innocent life" suggest otherwise and must be regarded with caution.

In our opinion, abortion should neither be forced upon anyone nor denied to any woman who is competent to decide with her physician whether to continue an early pregnancy that puts her at physical or emotional risk. A vocal and powerful minority in our society wants to make abortion illegal under most or all circumstances. Here are three questions for those who would ban abortion:

(1) Are they as concerned with the health and well-being of mothers and infants as they are with that of the fetus?

(2) Do they support education and effective family planning services to prevent accidental pregnancy and thus reduce the number of abortions?

(3) Do they believe that diversity of religious belief is to be welcomed and protected in our society?

If the answer is "yes" to these questions, we have much in common though we may still disagree about the permissibility of abortion.

For those who answer "no" to the first question, being born may have a greater value than living life. Some people (with support from some religions) feel that this life is unimportant, a brief moment in eternity, and that having the chance to have eternal life — by virtue of being born (perhaps being baptized)— outweighs other considerations, including the continuing life and health of the mother. We understand this point of view and respect its practice by those who subscribe to it, but it should not be imposed on others.

Those who answer "no" to the second question seem to link their stand against abortion with a stand against sex (at least sex that has no procreative goal). We agree that there is too much casual sex, "instant intimacy," and tawdry behavior around us, but "punishing" sex by prohibiting birth control doesn't work. There is plenty of evidence on this point.

If the answer to the third question is "no," then we are miles apart. We value religious freedom, and celebrate diversity of opinion and belief. Others have the right to argue in favor of one "true" religion, to proselytize, but in their zeal to save the unenlightened, they curtail the rights of some to worship as they choose. The pilgrims who settled this country risked their lives for this right, the one Thomas Jefferson thought was most important.

Psychology

- Are males and females psychologically different?
- Is homosexuality a choice?

MENTAL HEALTH

Sigmund Freud (1856–1939), the father of psychoanalysis, put sex at the center of psychology. But even he thought there was much more to psychology than sex, and once defined mental health as the ability to love and to work. See *Sigmund Freud: Exploring the Unconscious* by Margaret Muckenhoupt (Oxford, 1977).

Otto Rank (1884–1939), Freud's follower and later dissident, added the idea that mental health must include the ability to be both responsible and free, or cooperative and creative. In a democratic society like ours that values freedom, responsible self-government is the key. At the individual and family level, mental health is creative, responsible self-government. Rank also emphasized that privacy and self-definition go together, and that sex education often doesn't work because young people feel that outsiders (parents, teachers, preachers) are trying to invade or take over their most personal domain. See *Acts of Will: The Life and Work of Otto Rank* by E. James Lieberman (Univ. of Massachusetts, 1993).

HOMOSEXUALITY

Recent research suggests a genetic link to sex preference, that most people do not "choose" their sexual orientation, but instead inherit it. Of course, most genetic traits can be influenced by environment and experience — but the amount of influence may not be great. Through history, homosexuals have been persecuted, and have hidden their feelings. This is beginning to change.

An earlier insight on homosexuality comes from the British physician and sexologist Havelock Ellis. He wrote in *Psychology of Sex* (1933) that some homosexual men who were eager to change would, with the help of hypnosis, have intercourse with women. However, that would not change their basic feelings. One patient explained that it was simply masturbation with a female partner. For others, hypnosis failed entirely to change or "cure" homosexuality: "The subject resists the suggestion, just as the normal subject usually resists under hypnosis the suggestion to commit a crime." Books by Havelock Ellis are valuable still for what they say about "the facts of life" and more.

Sociology, Economics, and Politics

- Are teenage parents victims or villains in today's society?
- How are health education and health care affected by social forces?

Teen sexual activity has gone up over a generation but is beginning to go down slightly, while contraceptive use is increasing. The age at first marriage is up, so we can anticipate a decrease in divorce rates in the future (it is already down slightly, to an estimated 40 percent).

Birth control has been associated with eugenics — an attempt to decrease the reproduction of the less fit in favor of the fittest. This has been discredited as an aspect of elitist racism and classism. Genetic counseling is becoming more useful, and most people have similar views about the number of children they want. Privileged folks tend to realize those hopes more often than the disadvantaged: "The rich get richer and the poor get children."

One book that all students of the subject must know is Kristin Luker's *Dubious Conceptions: The Politics of Teenage Pregnancy* (Harvard, 1996). Luker, a sociologist, argues that teen pregnancy is more a symptom than a cause of poverty in our society, which used to "protect" girls from social ills, but now has "come almost full circle, pinning social ills on sexually irresponsible teens."

Ecology

- Is there a population problem?
- Should individuals factor ecology into their family planning decisions?

For a long time people worried that a nation's standing in the world, at least its ability to fight wars, would be threatened if its birth rate went down. Nowadays the reverse is heard more often. The most densely populated countries in our hemisphere, Haiti and El Salvador, already lack clean air and water. In Africa, Asia, and Latin America natural habitats, notably rain forests, are being destroyed at a rapid rate: People are cutting wood wherever they can find it to burn for fuel.

The United States has about six percent of the world's population but uses about 40 percent of its nonrenewable resources. It takes quite a few babies growing up in India to consume as much as one baby growing up here. Similarly, poor Americans do not "go through" as many pairs of shoes, motorcycles, cars, etc., as their more affluent countrymen. Therefore, efforts to stabilize population do not focus on a particular group, whether racial or economic, nor should they. We believe that stability will be reached by the rational choices of people in societies who can exercise informed consent for parenthood. For further information, contact Zero Population Growth. A good resource is *Elephants in the Volkswagen: Facing the Tough Questions About Our Overcrowded Country*, edited by Lindsey Grant (Freeman, 1992).

Women's Studies

Women have been judged good or bad, maternal or sexual, chaste or whorish for thousands of years. This has led to cruel practices, from chastity belts to witch trials to genital cutting. Medical authorities have encouraged some of these practices. Professions, after all, reflect the values of societies in which they are practiced. Even scientists are strongly influenced by the nonscientific beliefs they grow up with. There are many relevant resources, but one which includes a broad vista of history, sociology, and health is *For Her Own Good: 150 Years of the Experts' Advice to Women* by Barbara Ehrenreich and Deirdre English (Anchor/ Doubleday, 1978).

In *Reviving Ophelia: Saving the Selves of Adolescent Girls* (1994), psychologist Mary Pipher confronts the "junk culture" and other challenges awaiting youngsters at puberty. While focused on girls, the book has much to offer both genders, giving important insights into issues of personal development in a rapidly changing and often unsupportive world.

Math

- Can a girl get pregnant the first time she has sex?
- If the answer is yes, what are the chances?

If you answered "No" to the question, you would be right 96 percent of the time. Isn't 96 percent worth an "A"? No, it flunks. Why?

The egg released about every four weeks from the ovary can only be fertilized for a day or so. We can estimate that the average woman is fertile for about four percent ($\frac{1}{25}$), of the month. If a woman has unprotected intercourse on a random day, that is, without knowing whether an egg might be present, her chances of becoming pregnant are about four percent. To put it another way, if 100 women have unprotected sex on a random day, the chances are that only four will get pregnant from that one act. By the same reasoning, after only 12 such acts, about half the women will be pregnant (12 × 4 percent = 48 percent). It doesn't take long for a small percentage to multiply into a large number.

Why is contraception so important if the odds are only 1 in 25 of getting pregnant? Because pregnancy is such an important event, and because sex is a popular activity.

Would you take a ride with a friend who had a major accident "only" once for every 25 times he or she drove? Take airplane travel as another example: Would you fly on an airline that had "only" four crashes per 100 flights? You would not, nor would such an airline be in business at all. (There are 10,000 flights a day, and only a few crashes every year.)

Another example that takes some math to grasp: Unintended pregnancies occur frequently among women who use no contraception, and less often among those who use it. The latter group reflects the fact that contraception is not perfect for technical reasons and human fallibility. About 25 million U.S. women are sexually active but not intending to be pregnant. Four million use no contraception; 21 million do. The two groups contribute about equally to the number of unintended pregnancies, because the careful group is much larger, while the noncontraceptors are taking greater risks with sex.

Literature

• William Butler Yeats wrote: "But love has pitched his mansion in/ The place of excrement" ("Crazy Jane Talks with the Bishop").

What do you make of this statement?
- Discuss some poems with sexual themes: "Nelly Trim," by Sylvia Townsend Warner; "In the Interstices," by Ruth Stone; "To His Coy Mistress," by Andrew Marvell; "she being Brand" by e. e. cummings.

These and many others are found in *Erotic Poetry*, edited by William Cole (Random House, 1963). John Atkins, in *Sex in Literature* (Grove, 1970), has compiled a treasury of literary references to everything from kissing to dildoes, from "Stimulation by Word" to "The Lonely Pleasure" (masturbation). Presentations of sex range, of course, from the sublime to the ridiculous. Teachers and parents may need help from librarians in finding more of the former to compete with the latter, which dominate the magazines, movies, television, and newspapers surrounding us and our children.

Norman Kiell helps with his anthology, *The Universal Experience of Adolescence* (International Universities Press, 1964). A fine biographical resource on sexual initiation is *The First Time* by Karl Fleming and Anne Taylor Fleming (Simon & Schuster, 1975), including notables Maya Angelou, Art Buchwald, Erica Jong, Loretta Lynn, Benjamin Spock, and 23 others. The oldest contributor was born in 1884, the youngest in 1950, and the authors conclude that "the introduction to sex is about as complicated and difficult an experience as it has always been ... that men and women have had equal damage done to them, that in their hurts and hungers they are more alike than not."

Language and Communication

- Where do "dirty" words come from?
- Why is some knowledge "forbidden"?

In "Soap Operas and Sexual Activity: A Decade Later" (*Journal of Communication* 46 [1996]: 153–160) researchers Bradley Greenberg and Rick Busselle note that American teenagers are well-represented among the estimated 30 million adults who are regular viewers. The decade 1985–1994 showed an increased incidence of sexual incidents in soaps. Physical intercourse is featured more, involving primarily unmarried people, and with more visual emphasis. At the same time a substantial portion of the activity is portrayed with a negative emphasis, balancing "lust" with "disgust," and sex is rejected more than in the past by participants in the drama. Pregnancy and sexual responsibility get some attention, along with new themes such as date rape. The article can be a guide for a class study of content and trends in television and other media.

The F Word, edited by Jesse Scheidlower (Random House, 1995), is a serious and good-humored treatment of sexual slang. In *Forbidden Knowledge* (St. Martin's, 1996), Roger Shattuck includes a survey of sex manuals through history and observes: "The world teems with salutory influences and with poisonous influences. The critic's minimum responsibility is to recognize writings for what they are and to punctuate false claims" (289).

More academic but quite readable books on sexual language include *Medical Terminologies: Classical Origins* by John Scarborough (Oklahoma, 1992) and Isaac Asimov's *Words of Science* (Houghton Mifflin, 1959). These enjoyable works introduce etymology and create respect for our linguistic ancestors, especially Latin and Greek.

Appendix: Resources

The following organizations are excellent sources of information on adolescence, sexuality, birth control, teen pregnancy, sexually transmitted diseases and related topics. As time goes on, most organizations will have web sites. We list some outstanding ones here; they all have links to other related sites. Many will also be able to provide information on relevant CD-ROM, brochures and other materials.

Adolescence Directory On-Line (ADOL)
Indiana University
http://education.indiana.edu/cas/adol/adol.html
(Mental health, resources, teens-only page)

Advocates for Youth
1025 Vermont Avenue, NW, Suite 200
Washington, DC 20005
Tel:(202) 347-5700
http://www.advocatesforyouth.org
(Primarily teen pregnancy prevention)

AIDS Action Council
1875 Connecticut Avenue, NW
Suite 700
Washington, DC 20009
Tel:(202) 986-1300

Alan Guttmacher Institute
1120 Connecticut Avenue, NW, Suite 460
Washington, DC 20010

Tel:(202) 296-4012
http://www.agi-usa.org
(The leading research and information center on
   family planning)

**American Association for the Advancement of
   Science**
1200 New York Avenue NW
Washington, DC 20005
Tel: (202) 326-6400
http://www.aaas.org
(*Science Books and Films* reviews media for stu-
   dents)

**American College of Obstetricians and Gyne-
   cologists**
409 12th Street, SW, POBox 96920
Washington, DC 20090-6920
Tel:(202) 638-5577
http://www.acog.com

American Library Association
245 W. 17th Street
New York, NY 10011
Tel: (212) 463-6819
http://www.ljdigital.com
(ALA reviews media, makes recommendations)

American Social Health Association
P.O. Box 13827
Research Triangle Park, NC 27709
Tel: (919) 361-8400
National STD Hotline: 1-800-227-8922
http://www.sunsite.unc.edu/ASHA

Catholics for a Free Choice
1436 U Street, NW, Suite 301
Washington, DC 20009
Tel: (202) 986-6093

http://www.lgc.org/catholicvote
(Catholics supporting choice on birth control and
   abortion)

Center for Reproductive Law and Policy
120 Wall Street
18th Floor
New York, NY 10005
Tel: (212) 514-5534
http://www.crlp.org

**Centers for Disease Control and Prevention
   (U.S. Government)**
http://www.cdc.gov
   includes Youth Risk Behavior Survey, Maternal
   and Infant Health, and National Center for
   Health Statistics
National AIDS Clearinghouse:
   1-800-458-5231
   http://www.cdcnac.org

Coalition for Positive Sexuality
3712 North Broadway #191
Chicago, IL 60613
Tel: (773) 604-1654
http://www.positive.org/cps

Emergency Contraception Hotline
1-800-584-9911
http://opr.princeton.edu/ec/ec.html

HealthGate
http://www.healthgate.com

IYG
1-800-347-TEEN (evenings 7:00–10:00 eastern
   time)
(Peer support for gay, lesbian and bisexual youth)

Mothers' Voices United to End AIDS
http://www.mvoices.org
(Provides resources about sex and STDs and
  links to support groups)

**National Abortion and Reproductive Rights
  Action League (NARAL)**
1156 15th Street, NW
7th Floor
Washington, DC 20005
Tel: (202) 973-3000
http://www.naral.org

National Abortion Federation
1755 Massachusetts Avenue, NW, Suite 600
Washington, DC 20036
Tel: (202) 667-5881
http://prochoice.org

National Adoption Information Clearinghouse
330 C Street, SW
Washington, DC 20447
Tel: (703) 352-3488 or (888) 251-0075
http://www.calib.com/naic

National Campaign to Prevent Teen Pregnancy
2100 M Street, NW
Washington, DC 20037
Tel: (202) 261-5655
http://www.teenpregnancy.org

National Council for Adoption
1930 17th Street, NW
Washington, DC 20009-6207
Tel: (202) 328-1200

National Council on Family Relations
3989 Central Avenue, NE, Suite 550

Minneapolis, MN 55421
Tel: (888) 781-9331
http://www.ncfr.com
(Each year *Family Relations* reviews the best new videos)

National Family Planning and Reproductive Health Association
122 C Street, NW, Suite 380
Washington, DC 20001
Tel: (202) 628-3535

National Organization on Adolescent Pregnancy, Parenting and Prevention
1319 F Street, NW, Suite 400
Washington, DC 20004
Tel: (202) 783-5770
http://www.noappp.org

New York Online Access to Health (NOAH)
http://www.noah.cuny.edu

Planned Parenthood Federation of America
810 Seventh Avenue
New York, NY 10019
Tel: (212) 245-1845
Call: 1-800-230-PLAN to reach the health center near you.
http://www.plannedparenthood.org

Safer Sex
http://www.safersex.org/

SexQuest
New York University Human Sexuality Program
http://www.sexquest.com/

**Sexuality Information and Education Council
  of the United States (SIECUS)**
130 West 42nd Street, Suite 350
New York, NY 10036-7802
Tel:(212) 819-9770
http://www.siecus.org

Zero Population Growth
1400 16th Street, NW, Suite 320
Washington, DC 20036
Tel: (202) 332-2200
http://www.zpg.org

References

Of the many references cited, the following were most helpful in the overall preparation of this book: Hatcher, R.A., et al. *Contraceptive Technology* (16th Edition). New York: Irvington Publishers, Inc., 1994; Fact sheets from Advocates for Youth and the Alan Guttmacher Institute; Westheimer, R. *Dr. Ruth's Encyclopedia of Sex.* Continuum Publishing Co., New York: 1994; and E.J. Lieberman, E. Peck, *Sex & Birth Control: A Guide for the Young,* rev. ed. New York: Harper & Row, 1981.

Advocates for Youth. "The Facts: Adolescents, HIV/AIDS and other Sexually Transmitted Diseases (STDs)." Washington, DC: 1996.

_____. "The Facts: Pregnancy and Childbearing Among Younger Teens." Washington, DC: 1996.

_____. "The Facts: Adolescent Contraceptive Use." Washington, DC: 1995.

_____. "The Facts: School-Based and School-Linked Health Centers." Washington, DC: 1995.

_____. "The Facts: Adolescent Sexual Behavior, Pregnancy and Parenthood." Washington, DC: 1994.

Alan Guttmacher Institute. "Facts in Brief: Contraceptive Use." January 1996.

_____. "Facts in Brief: Teen Sex and Pregnancy." July 1996.

_____. "Facts in Brief: Induced Abortion." 1996.

_____. "Lawmakers Grapple with Parents' Role in Teen Access to Reproductive Health Care." *Issues in Brief,* November 1995.

_____. *Sex and America's Teenagers.* New York: 1994.

_____. "Facts in Brief: Teenage Reproductive Health in the United States." August 1994.

_____. "Facts in Brief: Sexually Transmitted Diseases (STDs) in the United States." 1993.

American Academy of Pediatrics. "The Adolescent's Right to Confidential Care When Considering Abortion." *Pediatrics* (1996), 97(5).

American College of Obstetricians and Gynecologists. "Barrier Methods of Contraception." Washington, DC: March 1995.

_____. "Birth Control." Washington, DC: March 1995.

_____. "Adolescents' Right to Refuse Long-Term Contraceptives." June 1994.

_____. Committee on Adolescent Health Care. "Safety of Oral Contraceptives for Teenagers." February 1991.

American Medical Women's Association. *Guide to Sexuality*. New York: Dell Publishing, 1996.

American Social Health Association. "Gallup Study: Teenagers Know More Than Adults About STDs, but STD Knowledge Among Both Groups Is Low." September 14, 1995.

Ammerman, S. "The Use of Norplant and Depo-Provera in Adolescents." *J. Adolescent Health* (1995), 16(5).

Bachrach, C.A. "Adoption Plans, Adopted Children, and Adoptive Mothers: United States Data, 1982." National Center for Health Statistics Working Paper 22, March 1985.

Benson, P.L., A.R. Sharma and E.C. Roehlkepartain. *Growing Up Adopted: A Portrait of Adolescents and Their Families*. Minneapolis, MN: Search Institute, 1994.

Boston Women's Health Book Collective. *The New Our Bodies, Ourselves*. New York: Simon and Schuster: 1998.

Catholics for a Free Choice. "Fact Sheet: Majority Report: Catholic Attitudes on Sex and Reproduction." Washington, DC.

Center for Reproductive Law and Policy. "Reproductive Freedom Facts: Emergency Postcoital Contraception." New York.

_____. *Reproductive Freedom in the States: Restrictions on Young Women's Access to Abortion Services*. New York: 1995.

Cohen, P. "The IUD: Birth-Control Device That the U.S. Market Won't Bear." *Washington Post*, August 6, 1996.

CONRAD. *1996 Annual Report*. Arlington, VA: 1996.

Consumers Union. "How Reliable Are Condoms?" *Consumer Reports*, May 1995.

Dave Thomas Foundation, Wendy's International. *Adoption Works ... for Everyone: A Beginner's Guide to Adoption*. Dublin, Ohio: 1992.

Female Health Company, Chicago, IL. "The Female Condom" (promotional materials).

Guttmacher, A.F. *Pregnancy, Birth and Family Planning*. New York: Viking Press, 1973.

Hatcher, R.A., et al. *Emergency Contraception: The Nation's Best-Kept Secret*. Atlanta, GA: Bridging the Gap Communications, 1995.

Hatcher, R.A., Axelrod, R., Sarah Cates, P. Levin and T. Wade. *Sexual Etiquette 101 ... and More*. Decatur, GA: Bridging the Gap Communications, 1995.

Hatcher, R.A., et al. *Contraceptive Technology* (16th ed.). New York: Irvington Publishers, Inc., 1994.

_____. *Contraceptive Technology: International Edition.* Atlanta, GA: Printed Matter, Inc., 1989.

Henshaw, S., K. Kost. "Abortion Patients in 1994-1995: Characteristics and Contraceptive Use." *Family Planning Perspectives* (1996), 28(4).

Himes, Norman E. *Medical History of Contraception.* New York: Gamut Press, 1963 [1936].

Institute of Medicine. *The Hidden Epidemic: Confronting Sexually Transmitted Diseases.* Washington, DC: National Academy Press, 1997.

_____. *The Best Intentions: Unintended Pregnancy and the Well-Being of Children and Families.* Washington, DC: National Academy Press, 1995.

_____. *Contraceptive Research and Development.* Washington, DC: National Academy Press, 1995.

Kisker, E. "Teenagers Talk About Sex, Pregnancy and Contraception." *Family Planning Perspectives* (1985), 17(2).

Lieberman, E.J. "Preventive Psychiatry and Family Planning." *Journal of Marriage and the Family* (1964), 26:471–477.

_____. "Leveling with Young People About Sex." *Journal of the American Medical Association* (1969), 210:711–712.

_____. "Informed Consent for Parenthood." In *Abortion and the Unwanted Child,* C. Reiterman, ed. New York: Springer, 1971, 77–84. Reprinted, *American Journal of Psychoanalysis* (1974), 34:155–159.

_____. "Teenage Sex and Birth Control." *Journal of the American Medical Association* (1978), 240:275–276.

_____. "Adolescent Pregnancy." In *Basic Handbook of Child Psychiatry,* J. Noshpitz, ed. Vol. IV, 66–68. New York: Basic Books, 1979.

_____, ed. "Changing Family Patterns." APA Task Force Report No. 25, Washington, DC, 1986.

_____, Peck, E. *Sex & Birth Control: A Guide for the Young* (rev. ed.). New York: Schocken Books, 1981.

McLaughlin, L. *The Pill, John Rock, and the Church.* Boston: Little, Brown, 1982.

McLaughlin, S.D., D.L. Manninen, L.D. Winges. "Do Adolescents Who Relinquish Their Children Fare Better or Worse Than Those Who Raise Them?" *Family Planning Persp.* (1988), Jan/Feb.

Moskowitz, E., B. Jennings. "Directive Counseling on Long-Acting Contraception." *American Journal of Public Health* (1996), 86(6).

National Abortion Rights Action League. "Abortion, Breast Cancer and the Misuse of Science." Washington, DC: 1996.

National Center for Health Statistics. "The 1995 National Survey of Family Growth." Hyattsville, MD: National Center for Health Statistics, 1997.

National Council for Adoption. "Hotline Information Packet." Washington, DC: 1996.

Office of National AIDS Policy. "Youth and HIV/AIDS: An American Agenda." Washington, DC: March 1996.

Planned Parenthood Federation of America. "Facts About Birth Control." July 1995.

Russell, C. "Venereal Diseases Rampant Among America's Teenagers." *Washington Post*, Health, November 26, 1996, 7.

Sacks, Stephen L. *The Truth About Herpes* (3rd ed.). Seattle: Soules, 1992.

Siwek, J. "Consultation." *Washington Post*, May 28, 1996.

Span, P. "The Test of the Times." *Washington Post*, September 30, 1996.

Stotland, N. "The Myth of the Abortion Trauma Syndrome." *Journal of the American Medical Association* (1992), 268(15).

Thabault, P., P. Carr. "Nonhormonal Contraception." *The Medical Care of Women*, P. Carr, K. Freund, S. Somani, eds. Philadelphia: Saunders, 1995.

Troccoli, K. *One Stop Shopping: The Road to Healthy Mothers and Children.* Washington, DC: National Commission to Prevent Infant Mortality, 1991.

U.S. Department of Health and Human Services, Public Health Service, National Institutes of Health, National Cancer Institute. "National Cancer Institute Fact Sheet: Risk of Beast Cancer Associated with Abortion." February 13, 1996.

U.S. Department of Health and Human Services, Centers for Disease Control and Prevention. "Update: Barrier Protection Against HIV Infection and Other Sexually Transmitted Diseases." *Morbidity and Mortality Weekly Review* (1993), 42(3).

Urban Institute. "The 1995 Study of Adolescent Males." Washington, DC: Urban Institute, 1997.

Westheimer, R. *Dr. Ruth's Encyclopedia of Sex.* New York: Continuum Publishing Co., 1994.

Zhang, J., G.A. Thomas, E. Leybovich. "Vaginal Douching and Adverse Health Effects: A Meta-Analysis." *American Journal of Public Health* (1997), 87(7).

Index